A Clinician's Guide to Discussing Obesity with Patients

Sandra Christensen

A Clinician's Guide
to Discussing Obesity
with Patients

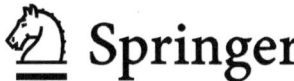 Springer

Sandra Christensen
Integrative Medical Weight Management
Seattle, WA
USA

ISBN 978-3-030-69310-7   ISBN 978-3-030-69311-4   (eBook)
https://doi.org/10.1007/978-3-030-69311-4

This Springer imprint is published by the registered company Springer Nature Switzerland AG
The registered company address is: Gewerbestrasse 11, 6330 Cham, Switzerland

To clinicians everywhere,

May your patients teach and inspire you as much as mine have taught and inspired me.

Preface

Obesity is the most common chronic disease in the United States with a prevalence that is growing across the globe. It leads to serious complications that significantly compromise health and increase mortality. The good news is that obesity is treatable, and treatment improves outcomes. When left untreated, it worsens. Yet despite its seriousness and the availability of effective treatments, it remains significantly undertreated.

Why is it that the majority of patients with obesity are not seeking or receiving effective treatment? The reality is that many of them do not know that obesity is a disease and that effective treatments are available. Even when they do view it as a disease, they believe that it is their responsibility to manage it. Unless their clinicians are starting the conversation and facilitating treatment, the situation is unlikely to change anytime soon. Despite the fact that obesity is the most common chronic disease in the United States, it is still uncommon for clinicians and patients to discuss it. This book was written to educate and inspire you to discuss obesity with your patients so that they can receive the treatment they need and deserve. Change starts with a single conversation between an informed clinician and a receptive patient.

As I write this, 42.4% of US adults have obesity and another 33% have a body mass index in the pre-obesity/overweight category, which means that over 75% of the adult population is an unhealthy weight. But it is not just adults; 19% of our children have obesity and the numbers are growing. Every time I contemplate or share these statistics with others, I feel a heaviness in my chest and a fire in my belly. The heaviness is the despair I feel at the prospect of these children and adults becoming increasingly unhealthy as obesity complications emerge and worsen. I am greatly concerned about the public health implications and see disaster ahead if we do not change the trajectory we are on. But I also feel a fire in my belly—a fire that has me doing everything I can to educate clinicians, alert policy makers, and teach people living with obesity that obesity is a serious, chronic disease and that effective treatment is available.

As a speaker and mentor, I regularly encounter clinicians who are passionate about learning how to treat obesity. Many are in busy primary care practices and want to know how they can help their patients lose weight and improve their health. They know that they have much to learn and recognize how important it is that they get started, yet do not know where to begin. I encourage them to seek education and point them to credible sources and organizations. Once they understand the pathophysiology and treatment approach, I move the conversation to weight bias and stigma, which are at the heart of why clinicians and patients are not talking candidly about obesity, and why obesity treatment is not often covered by insurance.

Over and over again, I witness the shame and internalized bias that my patients with obesity are plagued by and how profoundly it affects their physical and emotional health. These experiences have moved me to speak out against the harmful effects of weight bias and stigmatization for well over a decade. But it was not until I dove deeper into the literature about bias and stigma that I came face-to-face with the full extent of the damage. I was shocked at the sheer volume of research documenting the deleterious effects and the extent to which bias, stigma, and discrimination can infiltrate every aspect of a person's life. My heart broke open again and again, at times preventing me from researching and writing.

At the same time, racial unrest was arising in the country. Racial injustices were being broadcast and protested graphically and fervently with the goal of bringing about systemic change. I became acutely aware that racial discrimination and weight discrimination are not separate issues but are part of the same problem—a lack of education and a lack of commitment to treating all people with dignity and respect. This points to the need for individuals and systems to bravely look within to identify and eradicate bias and discrimination and create structures that support everyone.

But it was not just racial injustice that was in the spotlight while I wrote. The world was reeling from the COVID-19 pandemic. As more people became sick and the death toll rose, clinicians and researchers observed that those with underlying health conditions, one of which was obesity, were at greater risk of serious complications and death. I knew then, more than ever before, that clinicians need to address obesity head on in order to reduce the risks of poor outcomes from this virus and any that might follow, not to mention the need to reduce all of the other health risks inherent in obesity. My conviction further ignited my passion and fueled my writing.

This book was written to be a guidebook for you as you embark upon addressing obesity with your patients. It has been organized in a manner in which you can easily locate the information you need to take the first step, and the next, and the next. It will expand your knowledge of obesity and lead you into addressing it with your patients in a manner that is effective and professionally fulfilling. It begins with the science about the pathophysiology and evidence-based treatment strategies so that you understand the disease that you will be discussing. It explores the barriers that you and your patients face so that you can navigate them and move into successful conversations. In addition to providing you with the science and evidence for the strategies suggested, there are numerous real-life clinical scenarios and conversations that show you how to do it. These examples demonstrate how to open the conversation in a variety of practice settings with different types of patients so that you are able to make verbal choices that encourage rather than shut down productive conversation. Most importantly, these conversations can be accomplished in just a few minutes.

Over the years that I have specialized in obesity management, I have had the honor and privilege of working with some of the finest clinicians in healthcare. These passionate, knowledgeable clinicians have shown me the power of what can be accomplished when we work together to raise awareness and teach others about the need for obesity to be treated as the serious, chronic disease that it is. My closest associations have been with my colleagues at the Obesity Medicine Association. It is there that I have received the finest clinical education from those who are deeply committed to educating clinicians, reducing weight bias, and advocating for access to evidence-based treatment. In recent years, more professional organizations have seen the need to expand their obesity education and I have had the honor of participating in some of their initiatives. Two organizations with an unshakeable commitment to obesity education are the American Association of Nurse Practitioners and the American Academy of Physician Assistants. Their educational offerings will do much to inspire and educate clinicians to treat and lead in the field of obesity medicine.

I have mentored clinicians who have inspired and delighted me. From the moment of our first contact, they have impressed me with their passion and commitment to treating obesity. Some have become leaders in the obesity field and are not only improving the health of their patients, they are teaching and leading other clinicians, who are following their lead and doing the same. Each one of them is sending out roots that continue to branch out, building a solid foundation for further growth. Their inspiring brilliance deepens my conviction to teach and mentor as many clinicians as possible.

That brings me to you. Your patients need you to bring up the topic of obesity and to introduce them to the possibility that it can be managed successfully. They need to know that you are their ally, not someone to be avoided. This may require you to release old approaches and embrace new ones that are more effective and provide a counternarrative to what they have been told and have now internalized. As you approach your patients with obesity, I encourage you to shed your preconceived and culturally inflicted beliefs about the people who are living with it. What I know for sure is that significant progress can be made when we reduce and eliminate the bias, stigmatization, and discrimination that are directed at those with obesity. It is truly the key to opening the doors to effective treatment for the millions of people who need it. My hope is that this book will inspire you to give your patients what they need to trust you, so that they will return again and again for the healthcare that they need and deserve.

Seattle, WA, USA   Sandra Christensen
January 2021

Contents

About the Author

Sandra Christensen is a board-certified nurse practitioner and has specialized in obesity treatment since 2005. She owns Integrative Medical Weight Management in Seattle, Washington, where she provides personalized, comprehensive obesity treatment. She is a fellow of the Obesity Medicine Association (OMA) and serves as a trustee on the OMA Board of Trustees. She is a contributing author of the OMA Obesity Algorithm and earned the Certificate of Advanced Education in Obesity Medicine from the OMA.

Sandra Christensen speaks on the topic of obesity at national, state, and local conferences and webinars and is involved in projects and initiatives that educate clinicians about obesity treatment and advocate for access to care. She is passionate about educating clinicians about the complexities of obesity. Through clinical practice, speaking, writing, mentoring, and advocacy, she empowers clinicians to address obesity with knowledge and compassion.

Chapter 1
Recognizing Obesity as a Disease

1.1 Introduction

Obesity is a global health concern that affects over 650 million adults worldwide. With another 1.6 billion who have pre-obesity/overweight, nearly one-third of the world's population is an unhealthy weight [1]. Obesity is the most common chronic disease in the United States with 42.4% of adults [2] and 18.5% of children under the age of 18 [3] living with the disease. An additional 33% adults are classified as having pre-obesity/overweight [3], which means that over 75% of U.S. adults are an unhealthy weight. Given that obesity leads to serious health conditions and shortens lifespan, it is imperative that clinicians in every clinical setting discuss and address it with their patients. But before clinicians can initiate productive discussions about obesity, they need a clear understanding of obesity—its causes, pathophysiology, diagnosis, and treatment—and how it affects the health of their patients.

1.2 Obesity Is a Disease

The first official recognition that obesity is a disease came from the World Health Organization in 1997 when it published *Obesity: Preventing and Managing the Global Epidemic* [4]. This groundbreaking publication identified obesity as a complex, multi-factorial, chronic disease that affects persons across the lifespan and cited the health consequences of not treating it as such. This report declared that obesity is a population problem, rather than an individual problem, and called for a systematic approach to developing preventative and therapeutic strategies to address the growing worldwide health crisis.

However, it was not until 2013, when the American Medical Association (AMA) passed a resolution recognizing obesity as a disease that the concept began to gain traction [5]. The AMA declaration garnered sufficient attention that it increased

© Springer Nature Switzerland AG 2021
S. Christensen, *A Clinician's Guide to Discussing Obesity with Patients*,
https://doi.org/10.1007/978-3-030-69311-4_1

awareness and moved the healthcare system and society closer to confronting the seriousness of obesity. In the years that followed, several declarations were made including the Canadian Medical Association in 2015 [6] and the World Obesity Federation in 2017 [7]. The most recent proclamation occurred on July 3, 2020 when the German Parliament declared obesity a disease [8].

While these official recognitions have moved the needle forward, awareness of obesity as a disease is still too low. Many clinicians, healthcare systems, insurers, and policy makers have not grasped the importance of recognizing and treating obesity as a chronic disease, illuminating the need for education and advocacy so that the doors to treatment can open for the millions who are in need of it.

Despite worldwide recognition that obesity is a disease, many still cling to the outdated notion that obesity is a lifestyle choice and that a few simple changes will resolve it. But the science tells a different story—obesity is a serious, complex, chronic health condition that adversely affects health. According to the Obesity Medicine Association, "Obesity is a defined as a chronic, progressive, relapsing, multi-factorial, neurobehavioral disease, wherein an increase in body fat promotes adipose tissue dysfunction and abnormal fat promotes adipose tissue dysfunction and abnormal fat mass physical forces, resulting in adverse metabolic, biomechanical, and psychosocial health consequences." ([9], p. 9).

Obesity is diagnosed in the adult patient when the body mass index (BMI) is ≥ 30 kg/m^2 and is classified as Class I (BMI 30.0–34.9 kg/m^2), Class II (BMI 35.0–39.9 kg/m^2), or Class III (≥ 40 kg/m^2) based on BMI (Centers for Disease Control and Prevention, n.d.). Super obesity is diagnosed when the BMI ≥ 50 kg/m^2 and super, super obesity when the BMI ≥ 60 kg/m^2 [10]. For those of Asian descent, overweight is diagnosed when the BMI is ≥ 23 kg/m^2 and an obesity diagnosis is made at a BMI of ≥ 27 kg/m^2 [11].

1.3 Pathophysiology

Obesity is the result of a complex interplay of genetics and environment that manifests as the accumulation of excess adipose tissue that impairs health. Both genetic and epigenetic mechanisms contribute to susceptibility and the development of obesity. The mechanisms by which the body accumulates excess adiposity include genetic and developmental errors, infections, hypothalamic injury, adverse reactions to medications, nutritional imbalance, and environmental factors that may be social/cultural, immune, endocrine, medical, or neurobehavioral in nature. Epigenetic factors contribute to obesity in offspring and future generations [9].

Adipocytes function as endocrine glands that produce hormones which lead to widespread inflammation and influence metabolic and immune function throughout the body. As such, they are directly related to insulin resistance and contribute to many of the endocrinopathies that are related to the pathophysiology of obesity [12]. Adipocyte hypertrophy and adipose tissue expansion, particularly in the presence of abdominal obesity, contribute to alterations in adipocyte and adipose tissue endocrine and immune responses. It is these responses that contribute to the development of elevated blood glucose, high blood pressure, dyslipidemia, and other metabolic states that worsen health [9]. The anatomic changes created by fat deposition in organs and other areas of the body result in conditions such as Non-Alcoholic Fatty Liver Disease (NAFLD), cardiovascular disease, renal disease, among others. In addition to contributing to derangements in metabolic, endocrine, and immune function, the excess accumulation of adipose tissue exerts physical force on the body causing stress damage to other body tissues [9].

Weight and appetite are tightly regulated by multiple neuro-hormonal processes that involve adipose tissue, endocrine organs, gastrointestinal tract peptides, and the central and peripheral nervous systems [12]. The hypothalamus plays an instrumental role in energy metabolism, appetite regulation, and feeding behaviors [13]. When hypothalamic function is altered by genetic and environmental factors, obesity may develop and/or worsen.

1.4   Adverse Health Consequences

Obesity complications are the result of cellular and organ anatomic and functional abnormalities, pathogenic adipocytes, endocrine and immune dysfunction, and physical forces caused by stress on body tissues. As such, they are not simply risk factors or co-morbidities. They present serious threats to health [9]. Obesity is the root of 237 conditions that include some of the most common conditions found in clinical practice such as elevated blood sugar, elevated blood pressure, dyslipidemia, cardiovascular disease, non-alcoholic fatty liver disease, osteoarthritis, gastroesophageal reflux disease, female infertility, polycystic ovary syndrome, urinary stress incontinence, male hypogonadism, and cancer. Obesity is associated with the development of 22 types of cancer and is responsible for approximately 5% of the cancers found in men and 10% in women, making it the second most common preventable cause of cancer [9, 14].

1.5   Obesity Management

Given the serious nature of obesity and the threat it poses to current and future health, the most effective strategy is to treat obesity first. When obesity is treated as the primary health threat, complications are likely to improve or resolve, and the development of new complications may be prevented. As is the case for other serious conditions, outcomes are improved when clinicians intervene early.

The benefits of obesity treatment go far beyond weight loss. Goals of treatment are to improve health, reduce body weight, improve body composition, and improve quality of life. Obesity treatment is most effective when clinicians and patients shift from a weight-centric to a health-centric approach. A weight loss of 5–10%

provides clinically meaningful benefits with improvements to the anatomic, physiologic, inflammatory, and metabolic processes that occur with obesity. Given the pathogenic nature of adipocytes and the negative effects of the physical forces of adipose tissue on the body, treatment that is directed at the reduction of adipose tissue will contribute to the prevention, improvement, and potential resolution of obesity complications. Clinical improvements seen with weight reduction include improved glucose and lipid metabolism, reduced blood pressure, improved cardiac hemodynamic function, as well as improvement in conditions such as obstructive sleep apnea, osteoarthritis, polycystic ovary syndrome, and depression. Weight loss contributes to a reduction in obesity-related cancers, as well as an improved response to cancer treatment and a reduced risk of cancer recurrence. Due to the epigenetic transmission of obesity and metabolic risk, weight loss in child-bearing women and men may have a positive impact on the health of future generations [9].

Obesity treatment is most effective when it is framed as chronic disease management. As is the case with other chronic diseases, the objective is not to cure, but to improve health and function, improve quality of life, and prevent complications [15]. Treatment is more intensive until the disease is stabilized, then transitions to maintenance. Like other chronic conditions, obesity is characterized by periods of stability followed by relapses. Indicators of relapse are weight regain, the worsening of complications, and/or the appearance of new complications. When relapses occur, treatment should be intensified until stability is regained before transitioning back to maintenance [16].

Frequent follow-up improves adherence to the treatment regimen and is associated with better outcomes, including reduced weight, BMI, waist circumference, and systolic blood pressure [17]. An average of 16 face-to-face visits per year is associated with the best weight loss outcomes [18]. When obesity is stable, follow-up frequency can be reduced, but should be increased when relapses occur.

One of the major challenges of obesity treatment is managing the metabolic adaptation that occurs with weight loss. The body defends its weight and adiposity by increasing the appetite stimulating hormone ghrelin and decreasing hormones that promote satiety including leptin, insulin, peptide YY, cholecystokinin, and glucagon-like peptide 1 [17]. In addition to these hormonal changes, resting metabolic rate may be reduced by up to 15% [19]. When these adaptations occur, patients may experience more hunger and less satiety, which are likely to contribute to greater difficulty in adhering to the treatment plan, particularly eating. Even in cases where there is no change to the treatment regimen, weight loss may plateau, and weight gain may occur. When this occurs, clinicians need to intervene by modifying and potentially intensifying the treatment plan.

1.6   Evaluation

A thorough and targeted evaluation is one of the most important components of comprehensive treatment, as the information gleaned will guide the treatment plan. A thorough assessment includes a history, physical exam, and laboratory and diagnostic testing. The manner in which the clinician conducts the evaluation, particularly the history, lays the foundation for a trusting, collaborative partnership.

The purpose of the history is to identify the physical and psychological factors that have contributed to—or have resulted from—obesity. It includes a health history, weight history, review of systems, family history, socio-cultural history, assessment of support systems, as well as information about current eating, physical activity, and sleep patterns. The weight history identifies the factors that have contributed to weight gain and/or have prevented weight loss and elicits information about past efforts, successes, barriers, activities, and life circumstances that have affected weight. It should also include a review of preventative health screenings, as many with obesity delay healthcare appointments and screenings due to fear of being stigmatized [20].

An obesity-specific physical examination includes height, weight, BMI, blood pressure, heart rate, respiratory rate, and waist circumference. It focuses on identifying the presence and severity of obesity complications, as well as identifying any metabolic dysfunction or other issues that will impact health and treatment.

Laboratory and diagnostic testing are utilized to identify obesity-related complications, determine their severity, and establish a baseline from which health improvements can be measured. Adiposity-related labs include hemoglobin A1c, fasting lipid panel, a comprehensive metabolic panel with attention to fasting glucose, liver function, and kidney function, thyroid stimulating hormone, and vitamin D levels. Other tests may be warranted based on findings from the history and physical examination [9].

It is important to note that while BMI is a useful screening tool, it is not a true measure of adiposity and does not assess the physical, mental, or functional health of an individual. Further assessment such as waist circumference and body composition analysis may be needed to identify those with excess adiposity that threatens metabolic health, even when BMI does not fall in the overweight or obesity categories. Obesity staging systems can be utilized to determine the extent of the disease and inform decisions about treatment intensity [21].

1.7 Comprehensive Treatment

Given the chronic nature of obesity, a comprehensive, long-term treatment approach is needed. Effective treatment is individualized, patient-centered, and matched to the disease burden [16]. Comprehensive treatment utilizes five treatment modalities—nutrition, physical activity, behavioral therapy, pharmacotherapy, and bariatric surgeries and devices. The four pillars of treatment are nutrition, physical activity, behavioral therapy, and pharmacotherapy [9]. Bariatric surgery may also be added to the treatment plan, but it does not replace the four pillars. Implementation of the treatment modalities is best accomplished in a stepwise manner. While comprehensive lifestyle management is the cornerstone of obesity treatment, it is often insufficient [22]. Due to the numerous challenges of weight loss, metabolic adaptation, and the reality of weight regain, patients often require additional treatment modalities [23].

1.7.1 Nutrition

The most effective dietary interventions are those that are evidence-based, promote patient adherence, consider patient preference, and specify the quality and quantity of calories. A variety of nutritional plans are available and are chosen based on the individual needs of the patient. Consideration is given to the desired health and metabolic benefits of a specific intervention, as well as personal preferences, food availability, cost, cultural considerations, convenience, and likelihood of adherence [9]. Nutritional plans need to be continued long-term, although it may be necessary to modify or shift to another approach, particularly if there are health changes or weight regain.

1.7.2 Physical Activity

Physical activity improves the cardiovascular, mental, and musculoskeletal health of people with obesity. Benefits include improvements in body composition, blood glucose regulation, and dyslipidemia, and decreased blood pressure, insulin resistance, risk of certain cancers, mortality rate, dementia risk, pain, and depression [9]. For these reasons, it is an important component of a comprehensive treatment plan. However, the degree to which it contributes to weight loss varies from person to person. It may have little to no impact for some, while others may have a greater response [24]. Despite variability of response during the weight loss phase, routine physical activity is often needed to maintain weight loss [17]. For this reason, as well as the numerous benefits to current and future health, it is an important component of comprehensive treatment.

1.7.3 Behavioral Therapy

Providing strategies and support for the necessary lifestyle changes that are required to successfully manage obesity is one of the most important interventions in obesity treatment. Those with obesity are typically aware of the impact their lifestyle choices have on their health and weight but struggle with the challenge of establishing and sustaining healthy habits. Patients need support as they embark on changing long-standing habits and break free of societal norms that affect eating, physical activity, stress management, and sleep patterns.

Patient-centered, realistic goals assist patients in maintaining healthy behaviors over the long-term. Comprehensive obesity treatment requires people with obesity to bring attention to their eating, movement, and medication regimen throughout the day. Healthy eating requires meal planning, shopping, prepping, and cooking. In an environment in which convenient, processed, and ultra-processed foods are readily available, much attention must be given to ensure that the person has healthy options readily available in workplaces, at social events, and while traveling. Patients need support and encouragement to proactively plan, and in many respects, go against the current eating norms in society.

Many workplaces have become sedentary and far too often people spend their leisure time engaged in activities that require little to no movement. Technology has made it such that very little physical effort is needed to accomplish many of our daily tasks. Patients need coaching to find ways to add more movement to their daily routines in order to counter these habits and societal norms. Specific attention must be given to scheduling time for the physical activity sessions that are needed to improve health and reduce or maintain weight. Given the sedentary nature of many jobs, patients need coaching on the need to arise from their seats once per hour and move around, even for a few minutes.

1.7.4 Pharmacotherapy

Effective obesity treatment often requires pharmacotherapy. Not only is it important to assess the patient's current medications to determine if any are contributing to weight gain or are impeding weight loss and make appropriate changes, it is important to consider adding anti-obesity medications to the treatment plan. FDA approved anti-obesity medications are evidence-based tools that target specific physiology to improve the disease through mechanisms of action in the brain, gastrointestinal tract, and adipose tissue, and are most effective when they are part of a comprehensive treatment plan that includes nutrition therapy, physical activity, and behavioral counseling. Anti-obesity medications facilitate the management of eating behavior, slow the progression of weight gain and regain, reduce weight, and improve health and quality of life [9]. Agent choice is based on the desired metabolic and feeding effects, as well as contraindications, cost, and patient preference [16].

Anti-obesity medications can make it easier for patients to follow their nutritional plans by targeting hormonal influences that stimulate the hunger and cravings that make it more difficult to resist the temptations that are so prevalent in the environment. They may be the only therapy that counters the effects of the metabolic adaptation that occurs after weight loss, with its resultant increase in hunger hormones, reduction in satiety hormones, and reduction in resting energy expenditure that often drives weight regain [25]. Because obesity is a chronic condition, pharmacotherapy may need to be continued throughout the lifespan, which is how pharmacotherapy is utilized for other chronic conditions such as diabetes and hypertension [17, 26].

1.7.5 Bariatric Surgery and Procedures

The four pillars of treatment—nutrition, physical activity, behavioral therapy, and pharmacotherapy—may be insufficient for some patients. Bariatric procedures should be considered for patients with severe obesity, those who would benefit from the metabolic benefits that surgery can produce, and patients for whom significant weight loss is needed to restore function and improve health. All bariatric procedures should be performed at an accredited bariatric surgery center by an appropriately trained surgeon. It is important to remember that bariatric procedures are one component of comprehensive obesity treatment, not a replacement for it.

1.8 Summary

Current and future health are improved when obesity is recognized and treated. Given the numerous health consequences of obesity, the earlier clinicians intervene, the better the outcome. When obesity is treated first, other conditions improve or resolve. A modest loss of 5–10% improves health and quality of life and reduces risk of future complications. Obesity treatment is most effective when it is health-centric rather than weight centric.

References

1. World Health Organization. Obesity and overweight. 2020. https://www.who.int/news-room/fact-sheets/detail/obesity-and-overweight.
2. Hales CM, Carroll MD, Fryar CD, Ogden CL. Prevalence of obesity and severe obesity among adults: United States, 2017–2018. NCHS Data Brief. 2020;(360):1–8.
3. Hales CM, Carroll MD, Fryar CD, Ogden CL. Prevalence of obesity among adults and youth: United States, 2015–2016. NCHS Data Brief. 2017;(288):1–8.
4. WHO Consultation on Obesity (1997: Geneva, Switzerland), World Health Organization. Division of Noncommunicable Diseases & World Health Organization. Programme of Nutrition, Family and Reproductive Health. Obesity: preventing and managing the global epidemic: report of a WHO Consultation on obesity, Geneva, 3–5 June 1997. World Health Organization; 1998. https://apps.who.int/iris/handle/10665/63854.
5. American Medical Association. Recognition of obesity as a disease H-440.842. 2013. https://policysearch.ama-assn.org/policyfinder/detail/H-440.842?uri=%2FAMADoc%2FHOD.xml-0-3858.xml.
6. CMA Policy Base. Obesity as a chronic medical disease. 2015. https://policybase.cma.ca/en/permalink/policy11700.
7. Bray GA, Kim KK, Wilding JPH, World Obesity Federation. Obesity: a chronic relapsing progressive disease process. A position statement of the World Obesity Federation. Obes Rev. 2017;18(7):715–23.
8. The European Association for the Study of Obesity. German parliament recognises obesity as a disease. 2020. https://easo.org/german-parliament-recognises-obesity-as-a-disease/.

9. Bays HE, McCarthy W, Christensen S, Tondt J, Karjoo S, Davisson L, Ng J, Golden A, Burridge K, Conroy R, Wells S, Umashanker D, Afreen S, DeJesus R, Salter D, Shah N. Obesity algorithm eBook. Obesity Medicine Association; 2020. https://obesitymedicine.org/obesity-algorithm/.
10. Lemmens HJ, Brodsky JB, Bernstein DP. Estimating ideal body weight—a new formula. Obes Surg. 2005;15(7):1082–3.
11. Consultation WHOE. Appropriate body-mass index for Asian populations and its implications for policy and intervention strategies. Lancet. 2004;363(9403):157–63.
12. Poddar M, Chetty Y, Chetty VT. How does obesity affect the endocrine system? A narrative review. Clin Obes. 2017;7(3):136–44.
13. Timper K, Bruning JC. Hypothalamic circuits regulating appetite and energy homeostasis: pathways to obesity. Dis Model Mech. 2017;10(6):679–89.
14. Bhaskaran K, Douglas I, Forbes H, dos-Santos-Silva I, Leon DA, Smeeth L. Body-mass index and risk of 22 specific cancers: a population-based cohort study of 5.24 million UK adults. Lancet. 2014;384(9945):755–65.
15. Grumbach K. Chronic illness, comorbidities, and the need for medical generalism. Ann Fam Med. 2003;1(1):4–7.
16. Christensen S. Recognizing obesity as a disease. J Am Assoc Nurse Pract. 2020;32(7):497–503.
17. Eckel RH, Bays HE, Klein S, Bade HD. Proactive and progressive approaches in managing obesity. Postgrad Med. 2016;128(Suppl 1):21–30.
18. Jensen MD, Ryan DH, Apovian CM, Ard JD, Comuzzie AG, Donato KA, et al. AHA/ACC/TOS guideline for the management of overweight and obesity in adults: a report of the American College of Cardiology/American Heart Association task force on practice guidelines and the Obesity Society. J Am Coll Cardiol. 2014;63(25 Pt B):2985–3023.
19. Lam YY, Ravussin E. Analysis of energy metabolism in humans: a review of methodologies. Mol Metab. 2016;5(11):1057–71.
20. Sutin AR, Stephan Y, Terracciano A. Weight discrimination and risk of mortality. Psychol Sci. 2015;26(11):1803–11.
21. Sharma AM, Kushner RF. A proposed clinical staging system for obesity. Int J Obes. 2009;33(3):289–95.
22. Gadde KM, Martin CK, Berthoud HR, Heymsfield SB. Obesity: pathophysiology and management. J Am Coll Cardiol. 2018;71(1):69–84.
23. Ryan DH, Kahan S. Guideline recommendations for obesity management. Med Clin North Am. 2018;102(1):49–63.
24. Swift DL, Johannsen NM, Lavie CJ, Earnest CP, Church TS. The role of exercise and physical activity in weight loss and maintenance. Prog Cardiovasc Dis. 2014;56(4):441–7.
25. Greenway FL. Physiological adaptations to weight loss and factors favouring weight regain. Int J Obes. 2015;39(8):1188–96.
26. Apovian CM, Aronne LJ, Bessesen DH, McDonnell ME, Murad MH, Pagotto U, et al. Pharmacological management of obesity: an endocrine society clinical practice guideline. J Clin Endocrinol Metab. 2015;100(2):342–62.

Chapter 2
Recognizing Weight Bias

2.1 Introduction

Weight bias poses numerous health threats to people affected by obesity and is an important clinical concern. It is prevalent in all areas of society and infiltrates every aspect of life, including the workplace, educational institutions, personal relationships, social interactions, and healthcare [1]. The impact goes beyond hurtful comments and is at the heart of the prejudice, discrimination, and marginalization that people with obesity experience, all of which negatively affect their mental and physical health.

Weight bias and stigma are major contributors to why obesity is not fully recognized and treated as a disease, why obesity rates are rising, and why the health of people with obesity is worsening rather than improving. Weight bias is one of the primary reasons behind the lack of insurance coverage for medical obesity management, anti-obesity medications, and bariatric surgery, as well as the lack of obesity education provided to clinicians.

In order to effectively discuss obesity with your patients, you need to understand the impact that weight bias has on both you and your patients, as well as the setting in which you provide care, the healthcare system, and the world at large. You need to know and understand the public health implications of the systemic discrimination that people with obesity experience. All of these factors come into play when you are speaking with and treating your patients with obesity, regardless of the reason they are seeking care.

© Springer Nature Switzerland AG 2021
S. Christensen, *A Clinician's Guide to Discussing Obesity with Patients*,
https://doi.org/10.1007/978-3-030-69311-4_2

2.2   Defining Weight Bias

Weight bias is a bias against those who are perceived to carry excess weight [2]. It is based on false beliefs about the causes of obesity and negative beliefs about the people who have it. Weight bias includes negative attitudes, stereotypes, actions, and expressions that are harmful and lead to stigmatization. Once a trait has been stigmatized, it often leads to discrimination. This is the case for obesity, which is commonly and strongly stigmatized [3]. Weight bias falsely attributes the causes of obesity to behaviors which are seen to be under an individual's control, such as overeating, being sedentary, and personality characteristics rather than genetic or environmental factors. Common beliefs about people with obesity are that they are lazy, dishonest, unmotivated, unintelligent, unsuccessful, less competent, non-compliant, sloppy, lacking in self-discipline [4].

Weight bias may be explicit and intentional or implicit and unintentional and may be expressed in overt or subtle ways. Explicit bias and attitudes are known and reflect personal opinions and beliefs, whereas implicit attitudes lie outside of consciousness [5]. Explicit bias and attitudes may manifest in overt ways such as derogatory comments, harassment, exclusion, bullying. The beliefs underlying these behaviors are conscious and the actions are conducted with intent. In contrast, implicit biases operating outside of conscious awareness may be contrary to the attitudes one consciously expresses. Even so, implicit bias is a better predictor of prejudice and discrimination [6].

2.3   Prevalence

People with obesity experience weight bias, stigmatization, prejudice, and discrimination in multiple forms in many aspects of their daily lives. Weight bias and discrimination are prevalent in American society and infiltrate every aspect of life including the workplace, educational institutions, healthcare, the media, family and personal relationships, and daily social interactions (Obesity Action Coalition n.d.). According to the Obesity Action Coalition, "Obesity is a major issue and is the last socially acceptable form of discrimination in our society." Making explicitly derogatory comments and jokes about people with obesity is common in Western society, as is portraying them as lazy, gluttonous, and undisciplined. Having negative beliefs and attitudes towards them is more socially acceptable than explicit racism [3].

Women experience a disproportionate amount of stigmatization, which spans employment, education, healthcare, mental health treatment, the media, and romantic relationships. Those from racial/ethnic minorities experience further stigmatization. This gender disparity affects health, quality of life, and socioeconomic outcomes [7].

Children and adolescents are also burdened with weight stigma, and discrimination. Common sources are school settings, parents, and family members, with teasing and bullying being the most common manifestations [8]. The negative emotional consequences cause significant harm to children, are long lasting, and are carried into adulthood [9].

2.3.1 Workplace

Bias in the workplace influences hiring preferences, promotions, wages. It may precipitate employment termination. When applying for jobs, people with obesity may be perceived as having low self-discipline, poor personal hygiene, less ambition, lower productivity, low ability for supervisory roles, and may be more likely to be hired for roles that require little face-to-face contact. They are less likely to be promoted or recommended for promotion by their managers and have a lower chance of being hired in high level positions than equally qualified candidates who are not affected by obesity (Obesity Action Coalition n.d.). Women with obesity are more likely to be in low-paying jobs and may earn up to 12% less than women without obesity. Men are also paid less and are less likely to be in professional and managerial positions. Those with obesity are also more likely to be terminated, even when they have excellent performance and employment records (Obesity Action Coalition n.d.).

2.3.2 Education

Weight stigma is a significant problem in school settings from kindergarten through high school and extends into post-secondary education. For children and adolescents, weight-based bullying is common. A National Education Association study conducted in 2011 identified weight-based bullying as the most problematic form of bullying in schools [10]. Children also experience weight stigma from their teachers who have lower expectations regarding their physical, social, and academic abilities and make more negative assessments of their performance than they would for a child who does not have obesity [11]. This stigma may follow a child into higher education. For example, candidates with obesity who participated in in-person interviews for a graduate psychology program received fewer admissions than their counterparts without obesity despite similar credentials and equally or slightly more positive letters of recommendation. This happened more frequently for female candidates [12].

2.3.3   Media

The media both shapes and reflects society's narrative about obesity and the people who have it. The prevalent narrative is stigmatizing and damaging, with the underlying current that people with obesity make poor choices and are therefore responsible for their condition. People with obesity are significantly more likely to be portrayed in the media as headless, wearing ill-fitting clothing, eating unhealthy foods, and engaging in sedentary behavior [13]. These portrayals appear in a wide variety of media, including television shows, reality shows, movies, YouTube, and news coverage, including television, internet news sites, and print media such as newspapers [14].

Weight-related reality television shows such as *The Biggest Loser* dramatize and exploit society's stereotypes by depicting the show's participants as lazy, unmotivated, and to blame for their condition. They emphasize weight loss over health and push the narrative that weight loss is attainable, even if the methods are unhealthy, unrealistic, and dehumanizing [14]. These biased portrayals are inconsistent with scientific evidence.

2.3.4   Parents and Family

Interpersonal weight stigmatization occurs in families and has lasting effects. The most prevalent source of weight stigmatizing incidents for children with overweight and obesity is the family, including parents. In one survey of women who had obesity as children, 53% reported that their mothers demonstrated weight stigma towards them and 44% indicated that it came from their fathers [15].This stigmatization may have included bullying and teasing [8]. The emotional scars have long lasting effects, often continuing into adulthood [9].

2.3.5   Healthcare

Weight bias and stigmatization of patients with obesity in healthcare is common and well-documented [16]. There is a considerable volume of research and data that indicate that healthcare is rife with weight bias, stigmatization, prejudice, and discrimination and that biased attitudes and behaviors negatively affect the delivery and quality of care for patients with obesity. When patients with obesity encounter weight bias in clinical settings, it is far more than an unpleasant experience, it is deleterious to their physical and mental health.

In this section, we will discuss the sources and consequences of bias and stigmatization in healthcare. Whether you are a clinician or an educator, it's important for you to understand all sources of weight bias and stigmatization in the healthcare system, which include clinicians, educators, clinical staff, office staff, the built environment, and the healthcare system itself. If we hope to improve the care of patients with obesity, all members of the system must expand their awareness and facilitate changes that improve the experiences that people with obesity have in healthcare settings.

2.4   Sources of Bias and Stigma in Healthcare

2.4.1   Clinicians

Weight bias is rooted in false beliefs about the causes of obesity. For clinicians, it is the result of a lack of clinical education about the causes and development of obesity, reinforced by personal and societal beliefs. Healthcare providers have both implicit and explicit bias and attitudes towards patients with obesity. Both types of bias—explicit and implicit—may be automatically triggered when they interact with patients and may negatively influence their behavior towards their patients with obesity. There is considerable evidence that physicians, nurses, dieticians, maternity and gynecologic providers, psychologists, professionals who treat eating disorders, medical students, and other healthcare providers have strong negative views about people with obesity [3]. It is not uncommon for clinicians to stereotype patients with obesity as lazy, undisciplined, and weak-willed [4] and assume that they will be less compliant to treatment recommendations [17]. In general, clinicians are more likely to attribute behavioral factors as the cause and reason for the persistence of obesity than to factors that are beyond the control of the individual. Many clinicians may have low expectations that their patients with obesity can achieve or maintain weight loss and may see treatment as futile [17].

A sample of 2284 U.S. physicians found that respondents have strong explicit and implicit anti-fat bias and that their bias is as pervasive as it is in general society [18]. The researchers found that self-reported explicit attitudes were slightly stronger than implicit attitudes, indicating that physicians may believe that it is socially acceptable to openly express negative attitudes about those who carry extra weight. Anti-fat bias was present in these physicians regardless of their gender, but it was more prevalent in male physicians than females. Higher rates of bias were seen in those who do not carry extra weight and were more prevalent in those who were white [18].

Similar attitudes have been found in physicians in the United Kingdom, France, Australia, and Israel. One study of British physicians reported that the participants view people who carry extra weight as having reduced self-esteem, sexual attractiveness, and poorer health. They attributed overeating, physical inactivity, food addiction, and personality characteristics as the primary causes of obesity [19]. A study of general practitioners (GPs) in France had similar findings. Of the 600 GPs that participated, 30% felt that patients with obesity are lazier and more self-indulgent than people of normal weight, whereas 60% cited patients' lack of motivation as the most common problem encountered when treating patients with excess weight. They were more likely to believe that overeating was the primary cause of obesity and ranked it above genetic and environmental factors [20]. The findings from a study of 752 Australian GPs reported that the respondents' most common frustrations in weight management were that their patients were non-compliant and lacked motivation [21]. In a study of 510 family physicians in Israel, 31% felt that people with overweight or obesity are lazier than those of normal weight and 25% agreed that they lack willpower and motivation when compared to normal-weight individuals [22].

High levels of both implicit and explicit anti-fat bias have also been observed in clinicians who specialize in obesity treatment [23].

Clinicians providing maternity care such as physicians, midwives, and other healthcare professionals have demonstrated stigmatizing attitudes about women with obesity when providing prenatal, perinatal, and post-natal care [24]. These providers expressed discomfort, intolerance, and feelings of revulsion towards pregnant women with obesity [25, 26] and believed that these women lacked the necessary skills, awareness, and motivation needed to successful manage their weight [27]. Women receiving maternity care report negative interactions with their providers, finding them to be rude, angry, and abrupt, as well as not taking them seriously and not adequately responding to their needs [28, 29].

Nurse practitioners (NPs) attending a national conference participated in an investigator developed survey that assessed attitudes and beliefs about people with obesity. The data showed that these NPs perceived those who have overweight or obesity as "not as good as others, not as successful as others, not suitable for marriage, untidy, and not as healthy" [30].

Nurses report negative attitudes towards those with obesity, indicating that they view those with obesity as non-compliant, overindulgent, lazy, and unsuccessful. As a result of these attitudes, 31% state that they "would prefer not to care for individuals affected by obesity" with 24% agreeing that people with obesity "repulsed them", and 12% indicating that they "would prefer not to touch individuals affected by obesity" (Obesity Action Coalition n.d.). In a study of 398 British nurses, 69% attributed an individual's choices about food and physical activity as the cause of their obesity, while 33% cited a lack of willpower with food as the cause. Only 8.2% of the nurses believed that people with obesity are motivated to make lifestyle changes [31]. Brown and Thompson [32] found that nurses with lower BMIs had higher rates of negative perceptions about people with obesity. When these researchers studied the attitudes and beliefs of 15 primary care nurses towards obesity management, they found that these nurses were aware that obesity is a stigmatized condition and took care to avoid weight-based stereotypes. However, some noted frustration about patients being non-compliant and trying to find "the easy way out."

Dieticians and dietetics students also exhibit negative attitudes towards patients with excess weight. Registered dieticians report beliefs that obesity is caused by emotional problems and poor goal-setting and have low expectations that their patients will comply with their treatment regimens [33]. Dietetics students assume that patients with overweight and obesity have poor quality diets and health and that they are unlikely to comply with the treatment recommendations [34].

Past studies have shown that mental health professionals ascribe more pathology and negative attributes to patients with obesity than to average-weight clients, even with identical presenting situations, in addition to providing a worse treatment prognosis (Obesity Action Coalition n.d.). Mental health clinicians who treat eating disorders are not immune to weight bias. Those with stronger weight bias are more likely to express more negative attitudes about patients with obesity, attribute obesity to behavioral causes, and perceive poorer treatment outcomes when treating patients with obesity [35].

2.4.2 Clinicians-in-Training

A bias against people with obesity bias has been documented in clinicians-in-training. Students in clinical rotations and practicums are highly impressionable. When they encounter preceptors and other clinical staff exhibiting weight bias, they are more likely to internalize those beliefs and become perpetrators of weight bias and stigma themselves [36]. Clinicians-in-training observe peers, clinicians, educators making fun of, or making derogatory comments regarding people with obesity. One study showed that 50% observed it in their instructors.

This exposure to obesity bias during clinical and educational experiences enhances the potential that students will engage in biased and stigmatizing behaviors when they care for patients with obesity [37].

Medical students are a source of bias and stigma. In a survey of 4732 first-year medical students from 49 medical schools, 74% exhibited implicit weight bias and 67% exhibited explicit bias. The researchers found that the implicit bias scores were comparable to those reported against racial minorities, whereas explicit attitudes were more negative towards people with obesity than those towards racial minorities, lesbians, gays, and people experiencing poverty. Respondents who were male, had lower BMIs, and were non-Black, had higher rates of implicit and explicit bias [38]. Another study of 354 third-year medical students showed that 33% self-reported a moderate to strong explicit anti-fat bias and 39% had an implicit anti-fat bias, as measured by the Weight Implicit Association Test (IAT). Two-thirds of the students were unaware of their implicit anti-fat bias. Explicit anti-fat bias was more common in male students and no demographic factors were associated with an implicit anti-fat bias [39].

In one study, nurse practitioner students identified significant obesity bias in the clinic setting during their practicum experiences [37]. In addition to observing biases related to equipment and privacy, they encountered preceptors, preceptors' colleagues, and other clinical and office staff making negative comments or jokes about people with larger bodies, often in situations in which the comments could be overheard by patients. One student described the following experience "The author had watched a doctor shame a patient for gaining weight, get frustrated in front of a patient when the patient offers excuses for weight gain and cut a patient's appointment off when the provider did not feel that the patient was making an effort to move forward in the program" [37]. Nursing students also encounter clinicians discriminating against patients with obesity and report observing clinicians mock them during physical exams [40].

Another study looked at weight bias in advanced trainees from physician associate, clinical psychology, and psychiatric residency programs and examined their perceptions of treating patients with obesity, causes of obesity, as well as their observations of their instructors and peers exhibiting weight bias [41]. These students reported that 63% of their peers, 65% of health-care providers, and 40% of their instructors made people with obesity a target of negative attitudes and derogatory humor and comments. While 80% of the respondents felt confident about their ability to treat obesity, 33% believed that patients with obesity lacked the motivation to make the appropriate changes. Over one-third of the students felt frustrated with this perceived lack of motivation and 36% believed that patients were non-compliant with treatment recommendations. Greater frustration was expressed by those with higher weight bias, particularly those who believe that obesity is caused by behavioral factors [41].

2.4.3 Healthcare Environment

Healthcare environments are another place in which people with obesity face weight bias, stigmatization, and discrimination. Many healthcare settings do not have the capacity to adequately accommodate the bodies of those with higher BMIs or accurately assess their health. Office and clinical staff may engage in language and practices that contribute to patients with obesity feeling uncomfortable, embarrassed, shamed, or unwelcome. Whether these factors are intentional or unintentional, they are a manifestation of weight bias, stigmatization, and discrimination and they are noticed by patients who describe them as major barriers to utilizing healthcare [42].

Chapter 5 will address these factors and provide further guidance on how to create a physical and emotional environment in which patients with obesity feel safe, comfortable, and welcome.

2.5 Consequences of Bias and Stigma in Healthcare

Weight bias and stigmatization have numerous negative consequences for people with obesity. From compromised clinician-patient relationships to avoidance of routine and preventative care to a greater likelihood of engaging in unhealthy behaviors, weight bias and stigmatization have deleterious effects on the physical and psychological health of people who experience it.

2.5.1 Compromised Care

Quality of care and clinician decision making may be compromised due to weight bias and stigmatization. Disparities exist in the amount of time providers spend with patients with obesity as compared to those who do not have it. Primary care providers in one study indicated that they spend 28% less time than they do with their patients who do not have obesity and are more likely to consider the encounter a waste of time [43]. As a result, patients with obesity often get inadequate time with their providers [44] and many feel that their clinicians would prefer not to treat them at all [43]. Given the health complexities of obesity, patients often need more time with their providers, not less. People with higher BMIs are nearly three times as likely to say that they have been denied appropriate healthcare than those with normal BMIs [45].

Patients with obesity report that their clinicians often attribute their health concerns and conditions to their weight. When they present with concerning symptoms, patients with obesity are more likely to receive lifestyle recommendations or be advised to lose weight than they are to receive diagnostic testing, prescription medications, or be offered treatments than their counterparts without obesity [3, 17]. When clinicians attribute reported symptoms as being the result of excess weight, they run the risk that they will miss other conditions, some of which may be serious, and treatment will be delayed. One example is illustrated in the story of a patient who presented to multiple physicians over the course of 6 years with shortness of breath, coughing, hemoptysis, and coughing episodes so severe that she vomited or experienced urinary incontinence. Clinician after clinician told her that weight loss would resolve her symptoms and improve her immune system and rarely investigated further. She eventually found a primary care physician who took her seriously and after diagnostic testing and specialist evaluations, was diagnosed with lung cancer [46] [47].

Although women with obesity are at higher risk for gynecologic cancers such as endometrial and ovarian cancer, physicians have reported a reluctance to perform pelvic exams [48]. Given the increased risk of gynecologic cancers with obesity, these women need regular, thorough screening.

2.5.2 Compromised Clinician-Patient Relationships

A clinician's weight bias compromises the clinician-patient relationship on many levels. It not only damages the therapeutic relationship; it inflicts harm on patients.

Weight bias and the miscommunication that occurs between clinicians and their patients with obesity leads to a vicious cycle that ultimately worsens obesity and health [49]. Stigmatizing and discriminatory treatment is more damaging when it comes from influential people such as clinicians, making it all the more important that clinicians are able to recognize and reduce their weight bias in the clinical setting [47].

Primary care providers report less respect for their patients with obesity, which results in less positive affective communication and a tendency to be less forthcoming with information [50]. Physicians engage in less rapport building behaviors such as empathy, concern, reassurance, partnership, and self-disclosure with their patients with overweight and obesity. The relationship is weakened without this emotional connection, leading to less adherence to recommendations and decreased effectiveness of patient counseling [51]. Clinician communication is less patient-centered with those from stigmatized groups, including those with obesity [51]. When clinicians' explicit beliefs about obesity impair patient-centered communication, the result is mistrust of the clinician, less weight loss, and negative mental health outcomes [52–54].

Clinicians' negative views about their patients with obesity do not go unnoticed by their patients who are likely to feel disrespected, inadequate, and unwelcome [3]. In a study in which 2400 women with obesity were asked about their experiences with physicians, 69% indicated that their physicians were a source of bias and stigma. And 52% indicated that they had been stigmatized on multiple occasions (Obesity Action Coalition n.d.).

When patients feel stigmatized they are more likely to withdraw and less likely to fully participate in the encounter resulting in an inability or reduced ability to recall the advice or instructions of the clinician or adhere to the recommended treatment [3]. In one study, 70% of patients from two groups of patients—those seeking bariatric surgery and those enrolling in a clinical trial for an anti-obesity medication—believe that most physicians do not understand the difficulties of obesity [55]. Understandably, this negatively impacts the quality of the encounter and makes patients less willing to seek needed healthcare [3].

There are further disparities for people of color. Black adults with obesity are less likely to report that their providers explain things well or spend adequate time with them when compared to white adults with a normal BMI. Black adults who are overweight were also less likely to report that they got adequate time with their providers [56].

One study examined the likelihood of patients with obesity switching PCPs due to negative interactions [57]. Results showed that people with obesity were likely to change PCPs at a rate 52% greater than their normal weight counterparts, while those with pre-obesity/overweight were 23% more likely. They also saw that those with pre-obesity/overweight or obesity had more visits to the Emergency Department (ED) and concluded that the practice of frequently changing PCPs impairs continuity of care and increases utilization of healthcare [57].

2.6 Impact on Healthcare Utilization

People with obesity report that they avoid seeking healthcare out of fear that they will be stigmatized [58, 59]. Stigmatizing environments can contribute to anticipatory stress and acute stress reactions that reduce the quality of the encounter with the clinician and impact the patient's ability to engage with the clinician and process the information provided [47]. Those with higher BMIs have higher rates of experienced and internalized weight bias, which lead to greater body-related guilt and body-related shame. Both increase healthcare stress and lead to healthcare avoidance [42].

Due to fear of being stigmatized or receiving biased comments and actions, people with obesity may delay or cancel medical appointments such as annual wellness exams, routine follow-up, and visits for concerning symptoms such as pain, shortness of breath, and orthopedic issues, among others. As a result, these patients do not receive adequate screening for cancers and other conditions, or treatment before a condition worsens. When one considers that those with obesity are at increased risk for numerous adiposity-related complications, including cancer, the fact that they are receiving less healthcare is alarming.

Perceptions of biased treatment in healthcare settings lead many patients to be less engaged in primary health care services [42]. Women with obesity see their weight as a barrier to receiving appropriate healthcare. They cite disrespectful treatment, negative attitudes of clinicians, embarrassment at being weighed, the lack of adequately sized medical equipment, and clinicians commenting that they need to lose weight as factors that contribute to their decisions to delay healthcare. They report delaying cancer screenings such as clinical breast exams, pelvic examinations, Papanicolaou (Pap) tests, and mammograms despite feeling significant concern about cancer symptoms. As BMI increases, they are even less likely to have a Pap test [58].

If a patient suspects that the clinician will be frustrated or disappointed with the patient due to the patient's struggle with weight loss or adherence to the treatment plan, the patient is likely to cancel or not show up for appointments [60]. One study of 216 women identified their weight as a reason to delay or avoid preventative health care [61]. These women avoided making future appointments if they had gained weight since their last appointment and expressed a desire to avoid being weighed on the scale in their provider's office citing fear that the provider would admonish them to lose weight [61]. Another study of women at risk for heart conditions showed that 26% of the 1011 participants viewed a diagnosis of heart disease as embarrassing because people assume that they don't eat right or exercise. These women indicated that they delay or cancel healthcare appointments to give themselves more time to lose weight, even if they are needed to assess heart health. This was true across ethnicities and socio-economic groups [62].

2.7 Physical and Psychological Health Consequences

When patients with obesity encounter weight bias in clinical settings, it is far more than an unpleasant experience, it is deleterious to their physical and mental health. The evidence shows that weight stigma leads to physiological and behavioral health changes that are associated with worse metabolic health and increased weight gain [4, 63, 64]. These health effects come from the stigmatization itself, as well as the internalized bias that often occurs as the result of stigmatization. Both contribute to reductions in self-regulation and an increase of cortisol [47, 65], as well as psychological distress that triggers coping behaviors such as unhealthy eating, disordered eating, and avoidance of physical activity [66].

Several studies demonstrate that the internalization of negative weight-based stereotypes is associated with frequent binge-eating and a refusal to follow a healthy eating plan when compared to those who have not internalized negative stereotypes [4, 67]. Data gathered during the first months of the world-wide COVID-19 pandemic in 2020 found that young adults who experienced pre-pandemic weight stigma had increased vulnerability to the distress caused by the significant changes and upheaval in their daily lives, as well as increased maladaptive eating behavior [68].

2.7.1 Physical Consequences

Stigmatization contributes to a whole host of other negative health effects including increased risk of all-cause mortality [69] and worsened metabolic health [64]. For those who report weight stigmatization, the risk of dying is increased by 60%, independent of BMI [69]. The physiologic effects of weight stigma increase inflammation and disrupt metabolic processes resulting in higher C-reactive protein [70], an amplification of the relationship between abdominal obesity and hemoglobin A1c [71] and heightened cardio-metabolic risk [72]. The perception of elevated weight—even in those with a BMI that is not in the pre-obesity/overweight or obesity range—is associated with elevated blood pressure, C-reactive protein, cholesterol, triglycerides, glucose, hemoglobin A1c, and suppressed HDL [73].

A commonly held belief is that shaming people who carry extra weight will motivate them to lose weight [74, 75]. The evidence shows that the opposite is true. The stress of stigmatization triggers physiologic changes and behaviors that contribute to weight gain and increase the risk of obesity [4, 63]. Adults and children who self-report weight stigmatization have a higher risk of weight gain and of reaching a BMI in the obesity range that is independent of baseline BMI [76–78]. Patients who feel judged by their PCPs report difficulty with attempting and engaging in successful weight loss [79]. According to one study, those who perceive judgment from their PCP are significantly more likely to attempt weight loss but are less likely to achieve a weight loss of ≥10%, whereas those who do not feel judged are more likely to achieve it [79]. Patients with obesity are likely to feel shame due to repeated attempts to lose weight or maintain weight loss without success [80].

2.7.2 Psychological Effects

In addition to detrimental effects to physical health, people who experience perceived discrimination based on weight have mood and anxiety disorders at 2.5 times the rate of those who do not [81]. This effect has been seen in countries outside the United States, where depression risk is linked to elevated weight [82]. Studies show that poor mental health is the result of discrimination rather than the reverse [82].

Several studies correlate weight stigmatization with depression even after controlling for the effects of age, gender, age of obesity onset, BMI, physical activity, and binge-eating status [4]. Those with a history of weight-based teasing as children are particularly vulnerable to depression, indicating that negative childhood experiences related to weight continue to cause harm into adulthood. Adult bariatric surgery candidates reported that they had experienced weight-based stigmatization within the past month, including personal attacks [83], which was positively correlated to greater symptoms of depression [84]. In a large sample of adults ($N = 3353$) with a BMI $\geq$ 40 kg m^2, 40% reported that they have been mistreated due to their weight, which was significantly correlated with impaired mood [85]. In another study of women who have experienced frequent weight-stigmatization in childhood, adolescence, and adulthood, reports of higher depressive symptoms were reported [86].

2.8 Hope on the Horizon

Given the significant harm that weight bias, stigmatization, and discrimination cause, organized efforts to inform healthcare professionals, policymakers, and the public are occurring. In the *Joint International Consensus Statement for Ending Obesity Stigma*, a multi-disciplinary group of experts from around the globe speak out against the systemic stigma that damages health and undermines human and social rights, calling it unacceptable in modern societies [87]. This statement provides recommendations to eliminate weight bias and encourages academic institutions, professional organizations, media, public-health authorities, and governments to encourage education about weight stigma in order to facilitate a new public narrative about obesity.

2.9 Summary

Weight bias and stigmatization are prevalent in society and in healthcare and affect all areas of a patient's life. Weight bias is at the heart of why obesity isn't recognized and treated as a disease and contributes to the lack of access to evidence-based treatment. Healthcare is a common source of stigmatization, which compromises patients' physical and psychological health, and damages the clinician-patient relationship. Patients who experience bias and stigmatization in healthcare delay or avoid healthcare services, which has further negative impacts on their health.

References

1. Obesity Action Coalition. Understanding obesity bias brochure. n.d.. https://www.obesityaction.org/get-educated/public-resources/brochures-guides/understanding-obesity-stigma-brochure/.
2. Pearl RL, Puhl RM. Weight bias internalization and health: a systematic review. Obes Rev. 2018;19(8):1141–63.
3. Phelan SM, Burgess DJ, Yeazel MW, Hellerstedt WL, Griffin JM, van Ryn M. Impact of weight bias and stigma on quality of care and outcomes for patients with obesity. Obes Rev. 2015a;16(4):319–26.
4. Puhl RM, Heuer CA. The stigma of obesity: a review and update. Obesity (Silver Spring). 2009;17(5):941–64.
5. Phelan SM, Burgess DJ, Puhl R, Dyrbye LN, Dovidio JF, Yeazel M, et al. The adverse effect of weight stigma on the well-being of medical students with overweight or obesity: findings from a National Survey. J Gen Intern Med. 2015b;30(9):1251–8.
6. Greenwald AG, Poehlman TA, Uhlmann EL, Banaji MR. Understanding and using the implicit association test: III. Meta-analysis of predictive validity. J Pers Soc Psychol. 2009;97(1):17–41.
7. Fikkan JL, Rothblum ED. Is fat a feminist issue? Exploring the gendered nature of weight bias. Sex Roles J Res. 2012;66(9–10):575–92. https://doi.org/10.1007/s11199-011-0022-5.
8. Puhl RM, Peterson JL, Luedicke J. Weight-based victimization: bullying experiences of weight loss treatment-seeking youth. Pediatrics. 2013a;131(1):e1–9.
9. Puhl RM, Moss-Racusin CA, Schwartz MB, Brownell KD. Weight stigmatization and bias reduction: perspectives of overweight and obese adults. Health Educ Res. 2008;23(2):347–58.
10. Bradshaw CP, Waasdorp TE, O'Brennan LM, Gulemetova M. Teachers' and education support professionals' perspectives on bullying and prevention: findings from a National Education Association Study. School Psych Rev. 2013;42(3):280–97.
11. Peterson JL, Puhl RM, Luedicke J. An experimental assessment of physical educators' expectations and attitudes: the importance of student weight and gender. J Sch Health. 2012;82(9):432–40.
12. Burmeister JM, Kiefner AE, Carels RA, Musher-Eizenman DR. Weight bias in graduate school admissions. Obesity. 2013;21(5):918–20.
13. Puhl RM, Peterson JL, DePierre JA, Luedicke J. Headless, hungry, and unhealthy: a video content analysis of obese persons portrayed in online news. J Health Commun. 2013b;18(6):686–702.
14. Ata RN, Thompson JK. Weight bias in the media: a review of recent research. Obes Facts. 2010;3(1):41–6.
15. Puhl RM, Brownell KD. Confronting and coping with weight stigma: an investigation of overweight and obese adults. Obesity (Silver Spring). 2006;14(10):1802–15.
16. Alberga AS, Nutter S, MacInnis C, Ellard JH, Russell-Mayhew S. Examining weight bias among practicing Canadian family physicians. Obes Facts. 2019;12(6):632–8.
17. Persky S, Eccleston CP. Medical student bias and care recommendations for an obese versus non-obese virtual patient. Int J Obes. 2011;35(5):728–35.
18. Sabin JA, Marini M, Nosek BA. Implicit and explicit anti-fat bias among a large sample of medical doctors by BMI, race/ethnicity and gender. PLoS One. 2012;7(11):e48448.
19. Harvey EL, Hill AJ. Health professionals' views of overweight people and smokers. Int J Obes Relat Metab Disord. 2001;25(8):1253–61.

20. Bocquier A, Verger P, Basdevant A, Andreotti G, Baretge J, Villani P, et al. Overweight and obesity: knowledge, attitudes, and practices of general practitioners in France. Obes Res. 2005;13(4):787–95.

21. Campbell K, Engel H, Timperio A, Cooper C, Crawford D. Obesity management: Australian general practitioners' attitudes and practices. Obes Res. 2000;8(6):459–66.

22. Fogelman Y, Vinker S, Lachter J, Biderman A, Itzhak B, Kitai E. Managing obesity: a survey of attitudes and practices among Israeli primary care physicians. Int J Obes Relat Metab Disord. 2002;26(10):1393–7.

23. Tomiyama AJ, Finch LE, Belsky AC, Buss J, Finley C, Schwartz MB, et al. Weight bias in 2001 versus 2013: contradictory attitudes among obesity researchers and health professionals. Obesity (Silver Spring). 2015;23(1):46–53.

24. Mulherin K, Miller YD, Barlow FK, Diedrichs PC, Thompson R. Weight stigma in maternity care: women's experiences and care providers' attitudes. BMC Pregnancy Childbirth. 2013;13:19.

25. Heslehurst N, Moore H, Rankin J, Ells LJ, Wilkinson JR, Summmberbell CD. How can maternity services be developed to effectively address maternal obesity? A qualitative study. Midwifery. 2011;27(5):e170–7.

26. Schmied VA, Duff M, Dahlen HG, Mills AE, Kolt GS. 'Not waving but drowning': a study of the experiences and concerns of midwives and other health professionals caring for obese childbearing women. Midwifery. 2011;27(4):424–30.

27. Furness PJ, McSeveny K, Arden MA, Garland C, Dearden AM, Soltani H. Maternal obesity support services: a qualitative study of the perspectives of women and midwives. BMC Pregnancy Childbirth. 2011;11:69.

28. Furber CM, McGowan L. A qualitative study of the experiences of women who are obese and pregnant in the UK. Midwifery. 2011;27(4):437–44.

29. Nyman VM, Prebensen AK, Flensner GE. Obese women's experiences of encounters with midwives and physicians during pregnancy and childbirth. Midwifery. 2010;26(4):424–9.

30. Ward-Smith P, Peterson JA. Development of an instrument to assess nurse practitioner attitudes and beliefs about obesity. J Am Assoc Nurse Pract. 2016;28(3):125–9.

31. Brown I, Stride C, Psarou A, Brewins L, Thompson J. Management of obesity in primary care: nurses' practices, beliefs and attitudes. J Adv Nurs. 2007;59(4):329–41.

32. Brown I, Thompson J. Primary care nurses' attitudes, beliefs and own body size in relation to obesity management. J Adv Nurs. 2007;60(5):535–43.

33. McArthur LH, Ross JK. Attitudes of registered dietitians toward personal overweight and overweight clients. J Am Diet Assoc. 1997;97(1):63–6.

34. Puhl R, Wharton C, Heuer C. Weight bias among dietetics students: implications for treatment practices. J Am Diet Assoc. 2009;109(3):438–44.

35. Puhl RM, Latner JD, King KM, Luedicke J. Weight bias among professionals treating eating disorders: attitudes about treatment and perceived patient outcomes. Int J Eat Disord. 2014a;47(1):65–75.

36. Jansen S, Desbrow B, Ball L. Obesity management by general practitioners: the unavoidable necessity. Aust J Prim Health. 2015;21(4):366–8.

37. Hauff C, Fruh SM, Graves RJ, Sims BM, Williams SG, Minchew LA, et al. NP student encounters with obesity bias in clinical practice. Nurse Pract. 2019;44(6):41–6.

38. Phelan SM, Dovidio JF, Puhl RM, Burgess DJ, Nelson DB, Yeazel MW, et al. Implicit and explicit weight bias in a national sample of 4,732 medical students: the medical student CHANGES study. Obesity (Silver Spring). 2014;22(4):1201–8.

39. Miller DP Jr, Spangler JG, Vitolins MZ, Davis SW, Ip EH, Marion GS, et al. Are medical students aware of their anti-obesity bias? Acad Med. 2013;88(7):978–82.

40. Keyworth C, Peters S, Chisholm A, Hart J. Nursing students' perceptions of obesity and behaviour change: implications for undergraduate nurse education. Nurse Educ Today. 2013;33(5):481–5.

41. Puhl RM, Luedicke J, Grilo CM. Obesity bias in training: attitudes, beliefs, and observations among advanced trainees in professional health disciplines. Obesity (Silver Spring). 2014b;22(4):1008–15.
42. Mensinger JL, Tylka TL, Calamari ME. Mechanisms underlying weight status and healthcare avoidance in women: a study of weight stigma, body-related shame and guilt, and healthcare stress. Body Image. 2018;25:139–47.
43. Hebl MR, Xu J. Weighing the care: physicians' reactions to the size of a patient. Int J Obes Relat Metab Disord. 2001;25(8):1246–52.
44. Bertakis KD, Azari R. The impact of obesity on primary care visits. Obes Res. 2005;13(9):1615–23.
45. Carr D, Friedman MA. Is obesity stigmatizing? Body weight, perceived discrimination, and psychological well-being in the United States. J Health Soc Behav. 2005;46(3):244–59.
46. Dusenbery M. Doctors told her she was just fat. She actually had cancer. Cosmopolitan. 2018. https://www.cosmopolitan.com/health-fitness/a19608429/medical-fatshaming/.
47. Tomiyama AJ, Carr D, Granberg EM, Major B, Robinson E, Sutin AR, et al. How and why weight stigma drives the obesity 'epidemic' and harms health. BMC Med. 2018;16(1):123.
48. Adams CH, Smith NJ, Wilbur DC, Grady KE. The relationship of obesity to the frequency of pelvic examinations: do physician and patient attitudes make a difference? Women Health. 1993;20(2):45–57.
49. Fruh SM, Nadglowski J, Hall HR, Davis SL, Crook ED, Zlomke K. Obesity stigma and bias. J Nurse Pract. 2016;12(7):425–32.
50. Beach MC, Roter DL, Wang NY, Duggan PS, Cooper LA. Are physicians' attitudes of respect accurately perceived by patients and associated with more positive communication behaviors? Patient Educ Couns. 2006;62(3):347–54.
51. Gudzune KA, Beach MC, Roter DL, Cooper LA. Physicians build less rapport with obese patients. Obesity (Silver Spring). 2013a;21(10):2146–52.
52. Armstrong MJ, Mottershead TA, Ronksley PE, Sigal RJ, Campbell TS, Hemmelgarn BR. Motivational interviewing to improve weight loss in overweight and/or obese patients: a systematic review and meta-analysis of randomized controlled trials. Obes Rev. 2011;12(9):709–23.
53. Fiscella K, Meldrum S, Franks P, Shields CG, Duberstein P, McDaniel SH, et al. Patient trust: is it related to patient-centered behavior of primary care physicians? Med Care. 2004;42(11):1049–55.
54. Wanzer MB, Booth-Butterfield M, Gruber K. Perceptions of health care providers' communication: relationships between patient-centered communication and satisfaction. Health Commun. 2004;16(3):363–83.
55. Anderson DA, Wadden TA. Bariatric surgery patients' views of their physicians' weight-related attitudes and practices. Obes Res. 2004;12(10):1587–95.
56. Wong MS, Gudzune KA, Bleich SN. Provider communication quality: influence of patients' weight and race. Patient Educ Couns. 2015;98(4):492–8.
57. Gudzune KA, Bleich SN, Richards TM, Weiner JP, Hodges K, Clark JM. Doctor shopping by overweight and obese patients is associated with increased healthcare utilization. Obesity (Silver Spring). 2013b;21(7):1328–34.
58. Amy NK, Aalborg A, Lyons P, Keranen L. Barriers to routine gynecological cancer screening for White and African-American obese women. Int J Obes. 2006;30(1):147–55.
59. Puhl R, Peterson JL, Luedicke J. Motivating or stigmatizing? Public perceptions of weight-related language used by health providers. Int J Obes. 2013c;37(4):612–9.
60. Kirk SF, Price SL, Penney TL, Rehman L, Lyons RF, Piccinini-Vallis H, et al. Blame, shame, and lack of support: a multilevel study on obesity management. Qual Health Res. 2014;24(6):790–800.
61. Drury CA, Louis M. Exploring the association between body weight, stigma of obesity, and health care avoidance. J Am Acad Nurse Pract. 2002;14(12):554–61.
62. American College of Cardiology (ACC) 2016 scientific sessions. Special topics intensive session 54. Presented April 3, 2016. www.medscape.com/viewarticle/861382.
63. Puhl R, Suh Y. Health consequences of weight stigma: implications for obesity prevention and treatment. Curr Obes Rep. 2015;4(2):182–90.

64. Puhl RM, Heuer CA. Obesity stigma: important considerations for public health. Am J Public Health. 2010;100(6):1019–28.
65. Schvey NA, Puhl RM, Brownell KD. The impact of weight stigma on caloric consumption. Obesity (Silver Spring). 2011;19(10):1957–62.
66. Vartanian LR, Shaprow JG. Effects of weight stigma on exercise motivation and behavior: a preliminary investigation among college-aged females. J Health Psychol. 2008;13(1):131–8.
67. Puhl RM, Moss-Racusin CA, Schwartz MB. Internalization of weight bias: implications for binge eating and emotional well-being. Obesity (Silver Spring). 2007;15(1):19–23.
68. Puhl RM, Lessard LM, Larson N, Eisenberg ME, Neumark-Stzainer D. Weight stigma as a predictor of distress and maladaptive eating behaviors during COVID-19: longitudinal findings from the EAT study. Ann Behav Med. 2020;54(10):738–46.
69. Sutin AR, Stephan Y, Terracciano A. Weight discrimination and risk of mortality. Psychol Sci. 2015;26(11):1803–11.
70. Sutin AR, Stephan Y, Luchetti M, Terracciano A. Perceived weight discrimination and C-reactive protein. Obesity (Silver Spring). 2014;22(9):1959–61.
71. Tsenkova VK, Carr D, Schoeller DA, Ryff CD. Perceived weight discrimination amplifies the link between central adiposity and nondiabetic glycemic control (HbA1c). Ann Behav Med. 2011;41(2):243–51.
72. Pearl RL, Wadden TA, Hopkins CM, Shaw JA, Hayes MR, Bakizada ZM, et al. Association between weight bias internalization and metabolic syndrome among treatment-seeking individuals with obesity. Obesity (Silver Spring). 2017;25(2):317–22.
73. Daly M, Robinson E, Sutin AR. Does knowing hurt? Perceiving oneself as overweight predicts future physical health and well-being. Psychol Sci. 2017;28(7):872–81.
74. Callahan D. Children, stigma, and obesity. JAMA Pediatr. 2013a;167(9):791–2.
75. Callahan D. Obesity: chasing an elusive epidemic. Hastings Cent Rep. 2013b;43(1):34–40.
76. Hunger JM, Tomiyama AJ. Weight labeling and obesity: a longitudinal study of girls aged 10 to 19 years. JAMA Pediatr. 2014;168(6):579–80.
77. Jackson SE, Beeken RJ, Wardle J. Perceived weight discrimination and changes in weight, waist circumference, and weight status. Obesity (Silver Spring). 2014;22(12):2485–8.
78. Sutin AR, Terracciano A. Perceived weight discrimination and obesity. PLoS One. 2013;8(7):e70048.
79. Gudzune KA, Bennett WL, Cooper LA, Bleich SN. Perceived judgment about weight can negatively influence weight loss: a cross-sectional study of overweight and obese patients. Prev Med. 2014;62:103–7.
80. Thomas SL, Hyde J, Karunaratne A, Kausman R, Komesaroff PA. "They all work...when you stick to them": a qualitative investigation of dieting, weight loss, and physical exercise, in obese individuals. Nutr J. 2008;7:34.
81. Hatzenbuehler ML, Keyes KM, Hasin DS. Associations between perceived weight discrimination and the prevalence of psychiatric disorders in the general population. Obesity (Silver Spring). 2009;17(11):2033–9.
82. Hackman J, Maupin J, Brewis AA. Weight-related stigma is a significant psychosocial stressor in developing countries: evidence from Guatemala. Soc Sci Med. 2016;161:55–60.
83. Friedman KE, Ashmore JA, Applegate KL. Recent experiences of weight-based stigmatization in a weight loss surgery population: psychological and behavioral correlates. Obesity (Silver Spring). 2008;16(Suppl 2):S69–74.
84. Sarwer DB, Fabricatore AN, Eisenberg MH, Sywulak LA, Wadden TA. Self-reported stigmatization among candidates for bariatric surgery. Obesity (Silver Spring). 2008;16(Suppl 2):S75–9.
85. Carr D, Friedman MA, Jaffe K. Understanding the relationship between obesity and positive and negative affect: the role of psychosocial mechanisms. Body Image. 2007;4(2):165–77.
86. Annis NM, Cash TF, Hrabosky JI. Body image and psychosocial differences among stable average weight, currently overweight, and formerly overweight women: the role of stigmatizing experiences. Body Image. 2004;1(2):155–67.
87. Rubino F, Puhl RM, Cummings DE, Eckel RH, Ryan DH, Mechanick JI, et al. Joint international consensus statement for ending stigma of obesity. Nat Med. 2020;26(4):485–97.

Chapter 3
Reducing Weight Bias in Healthcare

3.1 Introduction

Quality of care can be optimized for people with obesity through the recognition and reduction of weight bias in healthcare settings. Healthcare professionals, educators, and students, as well as clinical and office staff need knowledge about the prevalence and negative effects of weight bias, as well as effective strategies to reduce the stigmatization and discrimination that patients with obesity experience in healthcare settings. It is up to all members of the healthcare team to reduce the hurtful and demoralizing experiences that contribute to the alienation and humiliation of people with obesity. Clinicians are in a position to lead the way.

Because implicit bias can interfere with clinical assessment, decision making, and productive clinician-patient relationships, it is important to recognize and reduce your implicit bias so that your patient's health is not compromised by attitudes that are outside of your conscious awareness. Once you have identified and explored your own bias, you are in a better position to identify how it manifests in your patients, colleagues, the systems in which you provide care, and society at large. Without an understanding of how weight bias affects these entities, it will be more challenging to change the trajectory of your attitudes and behaviors and influence others to do the same. Given the prevalence of internalized bias among people with obesity, it is vital that you understand how it manifests in your patients so that you can help them identify and reduce their internal bias.

This chapter will provide you with validated tools which will help you identify your bias, and strategies to explore and reduce it. Clinical scenarios will illustrate some of the ways in which clinician bias manifests in clinician-patient interactions and demonstrates how to interact with patients in an unbiased manner. Additional clinical scenarios will demonstrate how patients' internalized bias manifests and how clinicians can respond in a manner that counters the internalized bias.

© Springer Nature Switzerland AG 2021
S. Christensen, *A Clinician's Guide to Discussing Obesity with Patients*,
https://doi.org/10.1007/978-3-030-69311-4_3

3.2   Recognizing Weight Bias

3.2.1   Step 1: Become Aware of Your Own Bias

In order to provide quality care to their patients with obesity, clinicians must identify and overcome their own implicit and explicit weight bias [1]. Without examining your beliefs and behaviors, you may unknowingly continue them, causing harm
to those to whom you have vowed to provide the finest of care. Implicit biases are
biases that you are unknowingly hiding from yourself, which is substantially different from being unwilling to identify or change your behavior. When you are able to
recognize your own bias, you are in a position to challenge your negative stereotypes and assumptions.

Because we have all been influenced by the beliefs and behaviors of the healthcare community and society, as well as our own experiences, we all have bias, even
those who treat obesity. By accepting that you have bias, you are in a better position
to reduce it. You may already be aware of your perceptions about those with obesity,
but there may be some areas you haven't yet identified. With time you will be better
able to recognize your biased thoughts and behaviors and shift to more inclusive
thinking. When you know and understand your bias, you can manage it. When you
don't, it will manage you, influencing your interactions in ways that are unintentionally harmful. The goal is to understand your own mind so that it doesn't interfere
with your clinical assessment, decision making, and ability to have positive relationships with your patients.

3.2.1.1   Exploring Your Bias

Picture someone with obesity and notice the thoughts and feelings that arise. Don't
judge your thoughts and assumptions, simply notice them with curiosity and compassion. The goal is to make contact with your explicit bias and allow your implicit
bias to rise to your awareness.

Once you have made contact with your initial thoughts and feelings, ask yourself
the following questions. Notice your answers with curiosity and compassion.

1. When I see or encounter people with obesity, what assumptions do I make
   about their:
   • Character
   • Intelligence
   • Employment
   • Socio-economic status
   • Work ethic
2. When I work with patients with obesity, do I make judgements about their:
   • Character
   • Intelligence
   • Health behaviors
   • Motivation and ability to engage in treatment

3. Do I enjoy working with patients with extra weight or do I dread it?
4. When I'm in a room with a patient with obesity, am I comfortable or do I want to exit as soon as possible?
5. How much eye contact do I make?
6. What is my body language?
7. What type of assumptions do I make about the origins of the issue they are presenting with?
8. Do I consider them to be worthy of receiving a thorough evaluation and treatment?

In your next encounter with a patient who carries extra weight, notice your first associations. Then observe your behavior and decision-making process. Do you notice any consistent reactions or themes?

Once you have identified your thoughts and assumptions, ask yourself where they came from. Again, do so with tenderness and compassion and avoid judging yourself.

1. Are they based on your actual interactions with people with obesity?
2. Were they taught to you by your family?
3. Have you been influenced by portrayals in the media or the comments of colleagues, friends, or others?
4. How has society's stigmatization of people with obesity shaped your beliefs and attitudes?
5. If you have obesity, do you have these thoughts about yourself? Like others with obesity, you may have internalized society's bias.

These culturally inflicted beliefs arise from a lack of knowledge and habitual thinking and behavior that is not challenged.

3.2.1.2   Tools for Assessing Weight Bias

There are several validated tools available to assess weight bias. These tools identify implicit and explicit attitudes toward those who carry excess weight and can be utilized by clinicians on an individual basis, in educational settings, or to generate group discussions. If used in a group setting, it is best to keep individual responses private and focus on discussion that increases awareness about biases and leads to behavior towards patients that is free of prejudice.

3.2.1.3   Weight Implicit Association Test (IAT)

The most well-known of these tests is the Weight Implicit Association Test (IAT). Several IATs have been designed by researchers at Harvard to identify and study implicit attitudes and stereotypes towards people based on a variety of characteristics including race, gender, religion, gender, sexuality, and weight. The Weight IAT is one that was specifically designed to uncover implicit weight bias and it is available online, free of charge. Using a timed association task, the Weight IAT will help you uncover your unconscious associations towards people with overweight and obesity. This test will indicate if you have a slight, moderate, or strong preference for people based on their weight. The data that is collected is anonymous and is publicly available for use by scientists, journalists, educators, and others so that they can better understand attitudes and stereotypes The Weight IAT has been used in research that measures implicit weight bias both prior to and after educational interventions that have been designed to reduce weight bias (Project Implicit, n.d.). The Weight IAT will help you uncover your implicit biases so that you can learn more about them and consciously adapt your behaviors towards those that are less biased.

The test can be accessed at

https://implicit.harvard.edu/implicit/selecttest.html . Scroll down to the button labeled "Weight IAT."

3.2.1.4   Explicit Weight Bias Tests

Several explicit weight bias tests are available. The *UConn Rudd Center for Food Policy and Obesity* provides a toolkit that provides information about weight bias, as well as information about these explicit bias tests.

The following link will take you to the tests, which are also listed below:

http://biastoolkit.uconnruddcenter.org/module1.html

- Anti-fat Attitudes Questionnaire (AFA)
- Anti-fat Attitudes Scale (AFAS)
- Anti-fat Attitudes Test (AFAT)
- Attitude toward Obese Persons Scale (ATOP)
- Beliefs about Obese Persons Scale (BAOP)
- Fat Phobia Scale—short form Universal Measure of Bias-Fat Scale (UMB-FAT)
- Weight Bias Internalization Scale (WBIS)
- Weight Bias Internalization Scale—Modified (WBIS-M)
- Stigmatizing Situations Inventory (SSI)
- Stigmatizing Situations Inventory--Brief (SSI Brief)

3.2.2   Step 2: Reduce Your Bias

3.2.2.1   Become Educated

As a clinician, the most important thing you can do is educate yourself about obesity. Research demonstrates that weight bias in clinicians and clinicians-in-training can be reduced through education [2]. Obesity education should include the etiology, health risks, effective treatment approaches, and the physical, psychological & social effects of weight bias, stigma, and discrimination. This paradigm will help you shed your preconceived and culturally inflicted beliefs about obesity and the people affected by it and replace them with knowledge grounded in science. By familiarizing yourself with the science of obesity and recognizing it as a disease, your mindset will naturally shift to approaching it as any other condition with which patients present. As you replace your biases with knowledge, you will automatically reduce them.

3.2.2.2 Obesity Education

Chapter 1 provides a framework on the science of obesity and how it can be treated effectively. If you would like further obesity education, there are numerous resources and clinical education offerings available. Table 3.1 provides the names and links of organizations that provide clinical obesity education. Other resources are likely available in your professional organization. Table 3.2 provides you with additional educational resources on weight bias reduction.

3.2.2.3 Reduce Your Exposure

Because so many of our attitudes and beliefs come from our culture, it is nearly impossible not to be influenced by them. That is why it is imperative that we maintain vigilant about limiting our exposure to stigmatizing, discriminatory influences.

Table 3.1 Obesity education resources

Name of organization	Link
Obesity Medicine Association	https://obesitymedicine.org/
The Obesity Society	https://www.obesity.org/
Obesity Action Coalition	https://www.obesityaction.org/
STOP Obesity Alliance	https://stop.publichealth.gwu.edu/
The Rudd Center for Food Policy and Obesity	http://www.uconnruddcenter.org/
Obesity Canada	https://obesitycanada.ca/
World Obesity Federation	https://www.worldobesity.org/
The European Association for the Study of Obesity	https://easo.org/

Table 3.2 Weight bias reduction educational resources

Source	Link
Preventing Weight Bias Without Harming in Clinical Practice	http://biastoolkit.uconnruddcenter.org/
Understanding Obesity Stigma Brochure	https://www.obesityaction.org/get-educated/ public-resources/brochures-guides/ understanding-obesity-stigma-brochure/
Weight Bias in Clinical Care	http://uconnruddcenter.org/files/Pdfs/CME%20 Complete%20with%20links.pdf
Weight Bias in Healthcare	https://4617c1smqldcqsat27z78x17-wpengine.netdna-ssl. com/wp-content/uploads/Weight-Bias-in-Healthcare.pdf

Once you have identified the societal sources of your bias—the media, friends, family, colleagues, etc.—you can go out of your way to avoid those that you can avoid and reduce your exposure to those that you can't. Avoid programming that portrays people with obesity as lazy, gluttonous, of poor intelligence and character, or any of the other negative stereotypes that are perpetuated by the media. If you hear friends, family, or colleagues express biased opinions about people of higher weight, share your knowledge about the true causes of obesity and explain the harm that is done by perpetuating the stereotypes.

3.2.2.4 Collaborate with Colleagues

Discuss your personal experiences and beliefs about obesity with colleagues who are knowledgeable or interested in learning more. Such discussion has been shown to reduce weight bias in healthcare providers [2]. This can be done informally or formally. Start a discussion with a colleague in your healthcare setting, someone you know from your professional organization, or a former classmate. Form a discussion group or journal club that meets in-person or virtually. Members of the group can take the Weight IAT or one of the explicit bias tests available prior to the meeting and discuss their experiences of taking the tests, as well as what they learned from their results. Given the plethora of journal articles on weight bias and stigma and its negative effects, there will be no shortage of articles to discuss if a journal club is formed. The reference list at the end of Chap. 2 and this chapter will give you some excellent articles for this purpose. There is also the option of forming an online discussion group through social media or other forums. Participants can discuss their experiences and strategies and provide support for others as they recognize, examine, and reduce their biases.

3.2.3   Step 3: Educate Others on the Healthcare Team

3.2.3.1   Clinicians

Initiate discussions with other members of the healthcare team including your clinician colleagues, clinical staff, office staff, students, instructors, preceptors, and administrators. While you don't have control over the opinions and attitudes of others, simply raising the topic will make implicit attitudes more explicit both to the individuals who hold the biases and to others on the team. When biases see the light of day, there is a much greater potential that they can be challenged and reduced. By opening the discussion, you will likely find allies who will join you in your efforts to reduce weight bias in your clinical setting. Organize a forum in which the team can discuss how weight bias is impacting the care of patients with obesity and how it can be reduced. Request or organize education on obesity and the detrimental effects of weight bias for the entire team.

3.2.3.2 Educators

If you are an educator, discuss the topic with your colleagues so that you can add obesity education and weight bias education to the curriculum. If there is no formal curriculum, discussing weight bias with students, instructors, and preceptors will have a positive impact. Provide a forum from which students can ponder and reflect on their clinical experiences and apply strategies to recognize and reduce their bias in their clinical practices. Your presence and support in this process will be invaluable to their current and future practices and to the patients they serve.

3.2.3.3 Obesity Competencies

Professional medical societies and educators have recognized the need to include obesity education in both undergraduate and graduate curriculum. Two groups have developed obesity education competencies with the goal of incorporating these standards into undergraduate and graduate programs for healthcare professionals.

The Obesity Medical Education Collaborative (OMEC) is an initiative that was formed in 2016 by 15 professional organizations for the purpose of promoting comprehensive obesity education in undergraduate medical education, graduate education, and fellowship training [3]. Using the six Core Competencies of the Accreditation Council for Graduate Medical Education, the OMEC group members developed 32 competencies across six domains, with evaluation benchmarks for each competency. This effort is expected to increase the competence of clinicians to assess, prevent, and treat obesity [3]. It is the intention of the supporting organizations to extend use of the OMEC competencies and benchmarks in nurse practitioner and physician assistant programs in the future. For more information on OMEC, visit https://obesitymedicine.org/omec/.

Another initiative, *The Provider Competencies for the Prevention and Management of Obesity*, was collaboratively developed by the Provider Training and Education Workgroup of the Integrated Clinical and Social Systems for the Prevention and Management of Obesity Innovation Collaborative. This workgroup had representation from a group of 23 professional organizations that represent healthcare providers, educators, and other groups to whom obesity education would matter. This collaborative developed a set of educational competencies that include ten core competencies and 23 sub-competencies on the prevention and management of obesity [4]. These competencies can be incorporated into the curriculum of schools and training programs, licensing exams, board certification with the goal of educating future healthcare professionals, as well as continuing education programs for those already in practice [4].

3.2.4   Step 4: Recognize and Reduce Your Patients' Internalized Weight Bias

3.2.4.1   Recognizing Internalized Bias

Clinicians who treat patients with obesity routinely observe the internalized bias of their patients. Once bias has been internalized, patients believe the messages they've received, leading to discouragement and self-blaming. Those with internalized bias may blame themselves for their obesity and for their failure to lose and maintain their weight loss even if they are following the treatment plan consistently. Many think that information about eating and exercise should be enough to successfully lose weight and don't recognize the need for additional therapies and support. As a result, they may withhold information about their lapses and difficulties with following the treatment plan due to the assumption that they must be doing something wrong. They may also hide difficulties so as not to disappoint the clinician or be blamed for their challenges.

3.2.4.2   Reducing Internalized Bias

One of the most effective ways to reduce internalized bias is to educate your patients about the complexity of obesity. This will facilitate their ability to recognize obesity as a chronic health condition, rather than a lifestyle choice or a personal failing. Information about the contributing factors and physiologic processes by which obesity develops and worsens is vital to their understanding of their health and their weight and will help them to process and release their internalized bias. With time they will begin to realize that it's not their fault and that many of the strategies they have been told by society and other healthcare providers about obesity management are simplistic, inaccurate, and misinformed. When you notice body language that conveys shame or hear their self-critical comments, gently but firmly remind them that they are living with a chronic condition and that they are not to blame for their difficulties in managing it. This will not be a one-time event. Internalized bias can seem intractable at times, so don't be surprised if you need to address it repeatedly. With time, it will lessen, although it may emerge again in times of stress. It is your responsibility to be a steady presence and bring them back again and again.

As a clinician you have the opportunity to be a vector of healing for your patients with obesity—both from their past negative experiences in healthcare and from the effects of their internalized bias—so strive to make your patient encounters positive and respectful. As you model this attitude, patients will internalize your positivity and respect, which will change the manner in which they relate to their struggles with their weight and health. When you witness the effects of internalized bias in your patients, move the conversation to higher ground through your compassion and presence. Your interactions will provide them with an example of the type of interactions they should insist upon with other healthcare providers, as well as family, friends, co-workers, and others. You will give them the strength to speak up if they are blamed, shamed, or dismissed by other clinicians and healthcare personnel as well as others in their lives.

3.2.5 Step 5: Put Your Knowledge into Practice

3.2.5.1 Commit to Reducing Weight Bias

Make a commitment to reduce weight bias in all of your encounters with colleagues, staff, and most importantly, with your patients. Pledge that you will treat your patients with obesity with dignity and respect. Be compassionate and knowledgeable about how to deliver better healthcare and lessen the negative effects of weight stigma. Assume that patients have had negative experiences with other clinicians and healthcare workers and seize the power you have to provide them with a different and healing experience, one that will benefit them now and in the future. Build your toolbox of bias reduction skills and use them frequently. Share your knowledge and skills with other healthcare providers and your patients.

3.2.5.2 Manage Your Weight Bias

Maintain an awareness of your weight bias. If you find that biased thinking or behavior has entered your clinical interactions, consciously shift towards your new skills and behaviors. Identify what you and your patients have in common, which will soften your stance and help you connect with their experiences. Striving to see your patients' struggles through their eyes will bring you back to a more grounded place. By doing this, you can turn less than ideal clinical interactions into ones that open the door to deeper relationships with your patients. If you find you have conveyed bias, apologize to your patient, and move to higher ground. Remember, if you don't manage your weight bias, it will manage you, often in ways that you never intended. And finally, remember that you are not alone in needing to manage your weight bias. It is a practice that all clinicians must do on a daily basis.

3.2.5.3 Practice Curiosity and Compassion

Acknowledge the challenges that obesity and its management present to patients, clinicians, the healthcare system, and society at large. It is a complex condition with no simple solutions. Recognize that your patient has likely tried to lose weight multiple times with varying degrees of success. If you and your patient are doing everything you know to do and aren't getting the desired treatment response, resist placing blame on either party. Instead, be curious about what other factors may be affecting the treatment response. Regardless of the weight loss outcome, maintain a positive relationship with your patient, as this will have the biggest impact on their current and future health.

Remember that many of your patients may have experienced weight bias and stigmatization since they were young children. This is all the more reason to reassure them that you are aware of what they have experienced and that you are on their side. Explain that your goal is to interact in a non-biased manner and that you will likely make mistakes in the process. Invite them to tell you when they don't feel understood by you.

3.2.5.4 Keep Your Mind Open

Don't assume that the presenting symptoms are related to weight by exploring other causes. Even if the condition is a result of extra weight, it is still a valid concern and needs to be addressed through treatment of the condition and/or weight reduction strategies. Don't get caught in treatment inertia—either treat or refer for obesity-specific care. And remember to treat your patients with obesity with the same respect and concern that you would for any other chronic condition.

3.3   Clinical Conversations

Now that you have a better understanding of weight bias and stigma and its deleterious effects, let's look at some short clinical conversations that demonstrate the weight bias of the clinician. Each scenario will provide you with the clinical dialogue and identify the bias that is conveyed.

3.3.1   Clinician Weight Bias

Scenario #1
A patient is visiting a new PCP with a complaint of hip pain.
    Patient: "In the last month my hip has been hurting more than ever. It's getting difficult to do things around the house and run errands."
    Clinician: "It hurts because you are obese. If you lost some weight it wouldn't hurt."
    Patient: "Okay I'll try that."
    The clinician ends the appointment by leaving the room.

3.3.1.1   Biases Conveyed by the Clinician

All of the patient's health concerns are caused by her weight. The clinician spent less time with the patient than he might if the patient had a normal BMI. It also appears that the clinician is uncomfortable being in the room with the patient. This clinician called the patient "obese" which is derogatory and not consistent with People-First Language.

> **Scenario #2**
> An established patient presents to his PCP for his annual exam.
>   Clinician: "Your weight is up 15 pounds from this time last year. You need to lose weight, or your health will suffer."
>   Patient: "I know I've gained; it's been concerning me. I've tried to diet, but I can't stick to it. Work has been so busy and stressful that I haven't had much time to time to cook."
>   Clinician: "I tell all my patients to go to Weight Watchers and join the gym. It all boils down to eating less and moving more."
>   The patient does not respond and waits for the clinician to move on to the next topic.

3.3.1.2   Bias Conveyed by Clinician

The clinician is operating from the assumption that weight loss is simple, which is not aligned with the science. This clinician is not acknowledging that the patient is already aware of his weight gain and is concerned about it.

> **Scenario #3**
> The patient presents to her PCP for a diabetes follow-up.
>   Patient: "I've been trying to lose weight, but nothing seems to work. I'm so frustrated. Can you help me?"
>   Clinician: "It's all about calories in and calories out. It's a simple equation. You must be eating too much and moving too little. If you try harder, you will lose weight. Just eat less and move more."
>   The patient looks down at the floor and says nothing.

3.3.1.3   Biases Conveyed by Clinician

Weight loss is simple, and the patient isn't trying hard enough.

3.3.1.4   Discussion

All of these interactions depict common experiences that people with obesity have with their clinicians. These clinicians were not knowledgeable about the science of obesity or the components of comprehensive treatment. As a result, they were not able to offer effective weight management strategies or provide follow-up treatment. They did not recognize or reduce their weight bias or notice that it was negatively impacting their interactions with their patients. They did not intervene when their patients withdrew from the conversation or displayed body language associated with shame. In scenario #1, the clinician's mind was not open to exploring the complaint of hip pain and dismissed it as being caused by weight. In scenario #2, the clinician provided unsolicited advice about the need to lose weight, without any inquiry as to the patient's perception or readiness. The clinician offered non-specific interventions that are not grounded in the science of obesity treatment. None of the clinicians practiced compassion or curiosity. Productive conversation was shut down by all the clinicians, making it less likely that the patients will return for follow-up, preventative, or routine care. All of these effects will have a negative impact on their patients' current and future health.

Now let's revisit these scenarios with clinicians who understand obesity and the effects of weight bias.

Scenario #1

A patient visits a new PCP with a complaint of hip pain.

Patient: "In the last month my hip has been hurting more than ever. It's getting difficult to do things around the house and run errands."

Clinician: "That sounds challenging. Tell me more about what was happening when the pain worsened."

Patient: "About three months ago I started walking 2 miles with my friend every morning before work. My hip got a little achier at first, but I could handle it. I figured if I kept walking it would go away. But one day it really hurt by the end of the walk and since then I haven't been able to go because it hurts too much. I thought resting it would solve it, but it's getting worse."

Clinician: "It's good to hear that you've been walking. Let's get to the bottom of this."

Patient: "Thank you. I really want this pain to go away. Besides, I want to get back to walking with my friend."

Clinician: "I support your goal. Let's talk more about the pain and then I'll examine you to see what's going on and what we can do to make you feel better."

3.3.1.5   Discussion

In this example, the clinician did not make the automatic assumption that the worsened hip pain was the result of obesity. He kept his mind open and initiated an appropriate diagnostic evaluation that will likely lead to appropriate treatment. His compassion for the patient's pain and reinforcement of the patient's commitment to engaging in health promoting behaviors strengthened their relationship. If this was the patient's first encounter with this clinician, she would likely return in the future. If this was the patient's established provider, it's easy to see why she returned. It is likely that she has a trusting relationship with her provider due to having received un-biased care from him in the past.

Scenario #2
An established patient presents to his PCP for his annual exam.
   Clinician: "I notice that you've had some weight gain in the last year. Would you be comfortable discussing this further?"
   Patient: "I know I've gained; it's been concerning me. I've tried to diet, but I can't stick to it. Work has been so busy and stressful that I haven't had much time to time to cook."
   Clinician: "It's good to hear that you are concerned about your weight as it has an impact on your health. Weight management is challenging, but important. Would you find it helpful to talk to a dietician about some options for healthy, convenient meals and snacks?"
   Patient: "Yes, that would be very helpful. I really don't want to keep gaining weight."
   Clinician: "I will refer you to a dietician who understands weight issues and will develop a personalized plan that works with your lifestyle. Would you be willing to come back to see me in two months to discuss how it's going?"
   Patient: "Sure."

3.3.1.6   Discussion

This clinician approached the patient with respect and the topic of his weight loss difficulties without judgement. Her easy manner put the patient at ease, and he opened up about his concern about his health. The clinician clearly understood the complexities of obesity and the need for a personalized, step-by-step approach, as well as the importance of regular follow-up. By offering a follow-up appointment at a specific interval, the clinician conveyed her support and offered her steady presence in this patient's weight and health journey.

Scenario #3
The patient presents to her PCP for a diabetes follow-up.

Patient: "I've been trying to lose weight, but nothing seems to work. I'm so frustrated. Can you help me?"

Clinician: "I'm sorry you've been so frustrated. Yes, I can help you. Weight management is complicated, and many people find the conventional advice to be ineffective. Given the complexities of weight issues, people often need the help of their healthcare providers."

Patient: "What a relief! I really have been trying!"

Clinician: "I believe that you have. Losing weight is far more challenging than people think it should be. I can refer you to an obesity specialist who will do a full assessment and give you a personalized plan. Would you be interested in that?"

Patient: "Yes! I didn't even know there were specialists available."

Clinician: "Many people don't. In fact, many healthcare providers don't know it either, just as they don't know the science about obesity and how to effectively treat it, which is frustrating for patients. I'm glad you asked me for help."

3.3.1.7 Discussion

This clinician acknowledged the patient's frustration and educated the patient about the complexities of obesity and weight management. She didn't tell her patient to try harder or offer simplistic solutions. The clinician was informed about obesity specialists and made a referral just like she would for any other health condition that she did not have the expertise to treat.

3.3.2 Internalized Weight Bias

We will now look at two clinical scenarios in which the patient demonstrates internalized bias, and the clinician recognizes and reduces it.

Scenario #1
A patient presents for an annual exam with his established PCP.

Clinician: "It's good to see you. How have you been?"

Patient: "Doing pretty well."

Clinician: "Do you have any concerns?"

Patient: "I've been gaining weight and am frustrated with myself. I know what to do, but I'm just not doing it."

Clinician: "I'm sorry to hear you've been frustrated. Weight loss is a challenging and many people have experiences like yours. Tell me more about what you think you should be doing."

Patient: "I need to cut my calories and stop snacking. I need to stick to three meals a day with nothing in between. It's not rocket science. I just need to do it."

Clinician: "It sounds like you are being hard on yourself. My guess is that if it was easy to limit eating to three meals a day and eliminate snacking, you would do it. What if it's not that simple?"

Patient: "What do you mean?"

Clinician: "I mean that it's more complicated than what you may think. There are likely other factors contributing to your weight gain, not just what you eat, and other factors that make it difficult for you to manage your eating. Many people blame themselves because they have weight issues, but it's actually a complex health condition, not a lifestyle choice. Because it's so complex, people often need the help of their healthcare providers. Would you be interested in talking more about how I can help you?"

Patient: "I didn't know all that. Yes, I'd like to talk more about it."

3.3.2.1 Discussion

This clinician heard the patient's self-criticism in both word and tone. She identified his belief that his weight issues were based solely on eating and that altering his eating was a simple endeavor. She recognized that the patient felt entirely responsible for his condition and that he was blaming himself for his failure to control both his eating and his weight. This is consistent with what is known about internalized bias in patients with obesity—they accept the blame, believe it's a personal choice, and may struggle with maladaptive eating.

Scenario #2

A patient presents for a follow-up on a knee injury with an orthopedic specialist.

Clinician: "How is your knee feeling?"

Patient: "It's slowly improving but it's still pretty painful, which is so frustrating!"

Clinician: "I understand your frustration. It's no fun to be in pain."

Patient: "Yeah, I think it still hurts because of my weight. Since I hurt my knee, I've been gaining weight."

Clinician: "That's understandable since you can't exercise like you did before."

Patient: "That's part of it, but there's more to it. Since this happened, I've been eating more. Even when I'm not hungry, I just keep shoving food into my mouth."

Clinician: "It sounds like the stress and inactivity are impacting your eating and you're struggling to manage it."

Patient: "It's because I don't have any willpower. Nobody's forcing me to eat. I'm the one who puts it in my mouth. I've had this problem before, but it's worse now. I don't get it, I'm already fat, I don't need to gain more weight. Why don't I just stop?"

Clinician: "I hear that you are feeling bad about your weight gain and are blaming yourself, but it's more complicated than that."

Patient: "I'm not sure about that. I'm doing it to myself... and I have no one to blame but me."

Clinician: "It's not uncommon for eating habits to change when there's been an injury and physical activity is limited. And it's not uncommon for people who carry extra weight to blame themselves for their condition and the challenges associated with it. Would you be interested in speaking with a dietician who can help you manage your eating? She understands weight issues and will work collaboratively with you to manage your eating while your knee heals. I think it would help."

3.3.2.2 Discussion

Regardless of whether or not the patient accepts the referral, the clinician has already intervened in a manner that is beneficial. He has recognized the patient's internalized bias in statements such as, "Nobody's forcing me to eat," and "I'm the one who puts food in my mouth," and "I'm doing it to myself...and I have no one to blame but me." His responses educated the patient about the circumstances that contributed to the weight gain and the difficulty managing eating. The clinician also spoke directly about the internalized bias with the statement, "And it's not uncommon for people who carry extra weight to blame themselves for their condition and the challenges associated with it." While it's highly unlikely that this intervention will fully eradicate the patient's internalized bias, it will loosen its grip and provide the patient with a new frame from which to see her challenges. By offering a referral to a provider who also understands obesity, the clinician not only provided an intervention that targets obesity and will likely prevent further weight gain, he offered another opportunity for the patient to have a positive experience with a clinician. His referral is the opposite of considering any intervention to be futile. All of this is much needed for a person with obesity and internalized bias.

3.4 Summary

The care of patients with obesity is optimized when weight bias and stigmatization are recognized and reduced in healthcare settings. All members of the healthcare team must be aware of the ways in which weight bias and stigmatization jeopardize the health of patients. Clinicians are in a position to lead the way by identifying, exploring, and reducing their weight bias and then educating other members of the team. Clinicians are in a position to recognize the manifestation of internalized bias in their patients and offer corrective experiences that reduce internalized bias and shame and strengthen the clinician-patient partnership.

References

1. Fruh SM, Nadglowski J, Hall HR, Davis SL, Crook ED, Zlomke K. Obesity stigma and Bias. J Nurse Pract. 2016;12(7):425–32.
2. Geller G, Watkins PA. Addressing medical students' negative bias toward patients with obesity through ethics education. AMA J Ethics. 2018;20(10):E948–59.
3. Kushner RF, Horn DB, Butsch WS, Brown JD, Duncan K, Fugate CS, et al. Development of obesity competencies for medical education: a report from the obesity medicine education collaborative. Obesity (Silver Spring). 2019;27(7):1063–7.
4. Bradley DW, Dietz WH, the Provider Training and Education Workgroup. Provider competencies for the prevention and management of obesity. Washington, DC: Bipartisan Policy Center; 2017. https://bipartisanpolicy.org/library/providercompetencies-for-the-prevention-and-management-of-obesity.

Chapter 4
Barriers to Discussing Weight

4.1 Introduction

Clinicians and patients face numerous internal and external barriers to discussions about weight in clinical settings [1]. Each barrier is a brick that layer by layer builds a wall, blocking clinicians and patients from having conversations that move patients towards better health. Some of the bricks can be removed by the clinician, while others require action from the healthcare system, insurers, and policy makers. Before dismantling the wall, it's important to explore and understand the composition of each brick. This will provide you with a deeper understanding of what gets in the way. After we have dismantled the wall, we will use the bricks to pave a new path.

4.2 Clinician Barriers

Many clinicians see it as their duty to address obesity but face numerous barriers to doing so [2, 3]. Barriers include lack of knowledge about obesity and its treatment, weight bias, low prioritization of obesity, lack of knowledge about effective communication strategies, fear of making patients uncomfortable, concerns about their own credibility, lack of time, and concerns about reimbursement. Many of these barriers are real, while some are perceived. Regardless of their origin, they present clinicians with obstacles that need to be understood and navigated.

4.2.1 Lack of Knowledge About Obesity

One of the biggest barriers is a lack knowledge about obesity and its treatment. It is difficult to have effective conversations and direct patients into appropriate treatment without knowledge about the condition that is being discussed. Clinicians are

© Springer Nature Switzerland AG 2021
S. Christensen, *A Clinician's Guide to Discussing Obesity with Patients*,
https://doi.org/10.1007/978-3-030-69311-4_4

aware of the negative health consequences of obesity, but don't always recognize it as a chronic condition that warrants a chronic disease management approach. Even when clinicians recognize that obesity is a disease, they aren't aware that effective treatment strategies are available or have any referral sources [3].

Without adequate obesity education, clinicians lack knowledge about assessment, counseling strategies, and behavior management techniques [4]. They have a limited knowledge of how to conduct appropriate non-surgical clinical obesity care and how to implement obesity treatment guidelines on nutrition, physical activity, pharmacotherapy, and intensive behavioral counseling [5].

Many aren't aware of the need to diagnose obesity and document it in the medical record, which only happens 55% of the time, even when there has been clinician-patient discussion about obesity [2]. Underdocumentation of obesity also occurs in inpatient settings, even when clinicians recognize it and understand the clinical implications of leaving it untreated [6]. Without a diagnosis, patients don't receive appropriate care, referrals, or follow-up.

In the absence of knowledge of the pathophysiology and complexities of obesity, many clinicians have simplistic notions about how to address it and are less likely to understand the need for specialized treatment. They aren't aware that the specialty of obesity medicine exists and don't know about the components of comprehensive treatment. Because of this knowledge deficit, they view lifestyle changes such as healthy eating and regular exercise as the only effective advice and do not provide additional options for treatment. While they may recognize the benefits of bariatric surgery, they are much less likely to recognize that medical management, specialized nutrition, and behavioral counseling are warranted [2].

Without foundational knowledge of the etiology of obesity, treatment goals, and the health benefits of modest weight loss, many clinicians feel that treatment is futile. They are less likely to know that a loss of 5–10% confers numerous health benefits and significant risk reduction. When the erroneous expectation is that treatment is only successful if a patient achieves a BMI $< 25.0 \text{ kg/m}^2$, clinicians are much less likely to engage in discussion and treatment. When they are unable to view obesity through a chronic care lens, clinicians are more likely to be dismissive of anti-obesity medications, deeming them ineffective when their use results in a loss of 5–10%. They may also deem a modest weight loss from intensive lifestyle interventions as a failure, not recognizing the health benefits and risk reduction it confers.

4.2.2   Undergraduate and Graduate Programs

This lack of knowledge stems from a lack of obesity education in the undergraduate and graduate programs that prepare healthcare professionals for practice. Although it is changing, it is rare for students in physician, nurse practitioner, physician assistant, nursing, psychology, mental health, dietician, and nutrition programs to receive instruction that identifies obesity as a disease and outlines the current evidence on effective treatment.

A systemic review of obesity education from 2005 to 2018 found a paucity of obesity education for medical students, residents, and physician fellows throughout the world [7]. In order to ensure optimal treatment, obesity education needs to be included in undergraduate and graduate medical education [7]. Another study concluded that medical schools in the United States are not prioritizing obesity education in the curricula and are therefore not adequately preparing their students to manage obesity [8].

It is not just physicians that lack education, healthcare professionals with designations in nutrition, nursing, behavioral/mental health, exercise, and pharmacy also have a limited understanding of the causes of obesity [9]. With the exception of nutrition professionals, 78% of whom reported high quality training, these professionals were less likely to report adequate education in weight management—nursing, 53%; behavioral/mental health, 32%; exercise, 50%; and pharmacy, 47% [9].

Given that the majority of patients encountered in most clinical settings have pre-obesity/overweight or obesity and that many of the conditions that are being treated are caused by, or exacerbated by, excess weight, it is imperative that clinicians-in-training learn about obesity in their programs. Because knowledge about obesity is foundational to treating many of the conditions that will occupy many clinical hours in their future practice, inadequate obesity education places new clinicians in a compromised position when they begin their independent clinical practice.

Research indicates that inadequate obesity education is the result of inadequate faculty training. Faculty development is therefore essential to ensuring that clinicians-in-training leave their programs with the sufficient knowledge and skills to provide adequate obesity care [10]. Those who precept students in clinical practice sites also need to be educated about the diagnosis and treatment of obesity.

4.2.3 Continuing Education

Whether clinicians are new to clinical practice or are seasoned veterans, very little continuing education is available. Those who are interested must diligently seek it out. Some professional organizations have recognized the need and are dedicating more educational hours to it, but educational offerings for obesity are still just a smattering in comparison to the number of hours that are devoted to obesity complications such as cardiovascular disease, diabetes, cancer, and non-alcoholic fatty liver disease (NAFLD).

Lacking knowledge about evidence-based treatments, clinicians may have tried treatment and communication approaches in the past that were not successful. The frustration caused by these experiences may have been unintentionally translated into biases about their patients, which contributed to negative experiences for both parties [11]. This underscores the importance of providing obesity education, teaching strategies for effective conversation, and interventions that recognize and reduce clinician bias.

4.2.4   Professional Self-Efficacy

Many clinicians report low confidence in initiating discussions about weight and obesity [12]. Those who report low confidence cite a lack of knowledge about obesity as a primary reason. When clinicians have inadequate knowledge, they experience low self-efficacy in providing appropriate obesity, nutrition, and physical activity counseling to their patients [13]. Increasing clinicians' professional self-efficacy is regarded as the first step to improving obesity management [12].

4.2.5   Clinician Weight Bias

While it may appear on the surface to be a small and perhaps insignificant barrier, clinician weight bias is one of the biggest barriers for clinicians and may in fact be the biggest one they face. When a clinician views obesity as a lifestyle choice or moral failing and has negative beliefs about the person who has it, it is unlikely that the clinician will initiate a discussion that will be perceived as helpful by the patient. As outlined in Chap. 2, patients are deeply affected by the implicit and explicit biases of clinicians, making them less likely to return for screening, evaluation, and treatment, and less likely to initiate the discussion themselves.

As long as clinicians believe that obesity is the fault of the individual, very little progress will be made to improve the health of their patients with obesity. When less time is spent in appointments, fewer tests are ordered, and fewer interventions are performed, their patients' health will suffer. That's why every effort should be made to recognize and reduce clinicians' weight bias. As previously discussed, we all have weight bias, making it an ongoing task for all clinicians—even those who specialize in obesity—to recognize and reduce it.

Not using People First Language (PFL) when speaking with or about people with obesity is a form of weight bias that has profound negative effects on patients [14]. PFL for obesity puts the person before the disease and frames obesity as a condition the patient is experiencing rather than a label or identity. Referring to a patient with obesity as *obese* is the equivalent of referring to a person with cancer as *cancerous*. And the phrase *morbidly obese* is the equivalent of *morbidly cancerous*. While we all might understand how horrified people with a severe form of cancer would feel if they were called *morbidly cancerous* by their healthcare providers, we don't necessarily stop to think about how horrifying it is for a person with severe obesity to be called *morbidly obese*. In addition to the failure to use PFL, stigmatizing language is common among healthcare professionals and lessens the likelihood that patients will feel comfortable discussing weight with their clinicians [15].

4.2.6   Low Prioritization of Obesity

Clinicians may feel that there are more important clinical issues to discuss such as lipid levels or blood pressure control. This is confirmed by the Action Study, which found that 45% of clinicians feel that there are more important issues and concerns that need to be addressed before obesity can be discussed [2]. Clinicians may not recognize that obesity is often at the root of many of the conditions that need to be managed and therefore don't prioritize it. Their time is spent managing conditions that would improve if obesity were treated as the primary concern. As long as it is de-prioritized, patients will not get the clinical attention that is needed to success-fully manage their weight, and consequently will not achieve optimal outcomes for other weight-related conditions and complications. The best outcomes are seen when clinicians make it a priority to treat obesity first.

4.2.7   Lack of Obesity-Specific Communication Strategies

In addition to educational shortfalls about obesity, clinicians are not educated in how to initiate and continue productive conversations about weight. While they may be skilled at initiating conversations about other conditions, they may not be aware that there are specific techniques that should be utilized when discussing weight and obesity. Without an awareness of how patients may have been stigmatized in health-care settings in the past, they may not realize that conversations about weight and obesity need to be broached differently than conversations about other conditions. And once the conversation has begun, they may not know how to assess readiness and motivation before offering interventions [3]. And, as mentioned above, they may not realize the negative impact that commonly used phrases and terms such as *obese*, *morbidly obese*, and *fat* have on patients when they are used by their clinicians.

Fortunately, clinicians and other healthcare professionals are increasingly recogniz-ing the need for greater sensitivity and skill when communicating with patients about obesity [11, 16, 17]. In one study, nursing students reported that they lacked the confi-dence and techniques to discuss weight management with their patients and felt the need for advanced communication skills training in their nursing education [18]. The authors suggest that a lack of confidence and effective strategies may lead to avoidance of starting conversations about weight and weight management with patients.

4.2.8   Fear of Making Patients Uncomfortable

Because of the stigma associated with obesity, many clinicians are uncomfortable with candid conversation about it. Out of a fear of making their patients uncomfort-able, some clinicians don't broach the topic [3]. They may assume that their patients don't bring up the topic due to embarrassment about their weight [2]. Other assumptions are that the patient isn't interested, the patient isn't motivated, and clinicians' concerns about the patient's psychological issues and emotional state [2]. Clinicians may believe patients are aware of their weight and haven't been successful at managing it, so it's best not to bring attention to it. Clinicians who are aware of the impact of weight bias and stigma in the healthcare setting may fear that the patient will perceive their efforts as more of the same and that they won't be well-received despite their sincerity. Given these concerns, clinicians don't want to cause unnecessary pain. But this leaves clinicians in a quandary—they understand the importance of addressing this serious health issue but are afraid that raising the topic will add to the patient's distress and will ultimately be detrimental.

4.2.9   Credibility Concerns Based on Clinician BMI

People with obesity often feel stigmatized by their weight. This is true whether the person is a patient or a clinician. When you are the professional in the room whose role is to promote and improve health, it can be challenging to feel credible if you are struggling with the same condition, particularly one that is as mired in bias and misinformation as obesity. Clinicians are not immune to the effects of weight bias and may experience the same negative effects such as maladaptive eating, reduced physical activity, and psychological distress. Medical students with higher BMIs report implicit and explicit self-stigma and show higher levels of depression, anxiety, and substance abuse [19].

Some clinicians with obesity are concerned that patients will not find them to be credible and will not value the clinician's guidance or knowledge. Clinicians may imagine that patients are thinking, "Why should I listen to you?" or "What do you know about successful obesity treatment?" or "You obviously don't know how to help me if you don't know how to help yourself." This concern prevents clinicians with overweight or obesity from broaching the topic of weight with their patients. One study found that physicians with a normal BMI had a greater likelihood of initiating discussions about weight as compared to physicians with overweight or obesity [20]. When physicians perceived that their patients' BMI was equivalent to or greater than theirs, they were not only far more likely to initiate discussions about weight, they were also far more likely to record a diagnosis of overweight or obesity in the medical record. Physicians with a normal BMI were more confident about their ability to provide counseling on eating and physical activity to their patients with obesity than their colleagues with higher BMIs. The same study found that physicians with a normal BMI believed that patients with pre-obesity/overweight or obesity would be less likely to trust weight loss counseling from physicians with BMIs in the overweight or obesity range [20]. In addition to noting the increased confidence that is felt by physicians with normal BMIs, it suggests the possibility that clinicians with normal BMIs may be implicitly or explicitly communicating this bias to their higher weight colleagues, increasing the potential that these clinicians will internalize this bias and feel less credible about their ability to effectively counsel patients about weight issues.

While clinicians with normal BMIs may believe that they are more credible than their colleagues with higher BMIs, the evidence may suggest otherwise. In a study that examined the impact of PCPs' dietary advice on patients with pre-obesity/overweight or obesity found that while these patients generally trusted their PCPs, they trusted the dietary counseling they received from clinicians with higher BMIs more than the counseling that came from clinicians with normal BMIs [21]. This bias was also seen in a study of nutrition, nursing, behavioral/mental health, exercise, and pharmacy professionals, which found that when the clinicians' BMI was in the normal range, they were more likely to report success in helping their patients achieve clinically meaningful weight loss than clinicians with overweight or obesity [22]. An important difference in this study was that the professionals with higher BMIs did not report feeling less comfortable initiating discussions about weight or report less confidence in their ability to help their patients successfully manage their weight, nor did they perceive that their patients didn't trust their advice.

A study designed to reduce weight bias in teachers and student teachers through an online education intervention may provide further insights. Participants reported a higher prevalence of improved attitudes if the presenter carried excess weight as compared to presenters of a normal weight [23]. Although this study did not take place in a healthcare setting, the results suggest that when professionals are teaching others about weight and weight bias, a higher BMI may be an asset rather than a liability.

Although the evidence shows that clinicians with normal BMIs are more likely to believe that they are more credible at providing weight counseling to their patients, not all feel this way. Some have concerns that their patients will assume that the clinician doesn't understand obesity and can't relate to their struggles. Some patients directly ask clinicians if they have ever struggled with weight. When the answer is no, it is not uncommon for patients to tell clinicians that they feel too self-conscious about their weight to discuss it or enter into treatment with that clinician. These fears and experiences may deter the clinician from bringing up the topic with subsequent patients.

4.2.10 Lack of Time

One of the most daunting barriers is time. It is a large brick that blocks many conversations. Clinicians, particularly those in primary care, are already pressed for time. The time allotted for annual visits, problem-focused visits, and follow-up appointments are already shorter than what is needed. The thought of bringing up another topic feels impossible, especially one that needs to be handled as tenderly and thoroughly as obesity. Since it is rare for a patient to schedule an appointment for the sole purpose of discussing weight, the topic must be wedged into a visit that was scheduled to address a different health concern.

In the Action Study, lack of time was cited as a reason not to initiate a conversation 52% of the time. Even when clinicians are comfortable discussing weight, they don't believe they have the time to address it. And when it is discussed, only 24% of patients schedule follow-up [2]. Other studies confirm that time is a major factor in why clinicians don't bring up the topic [3, 24].

Another time concern is the fear that once the conversation begins, clinicians won't be able to keep it within the time allotted to the appointment, resulting in falling behind in their schedules. This is a valid concern, as once patients feel the space and safety created by their clinicians, they may open up in a way that is difficult to limit to the time available.

4.2.11 Reimbursement Concerns

The sad reality is that reimbursement for obesity treatment is poor in the United States. Very few insurers reimburse clinicians for obesity-focused visits. This has its roots in the bias and stigma that are associated with obesity and a lack of recognition that it is a disease that is as worthy of evidence-based treatment as other conditions such as diabetes, hypertension, and other chronic diseases.

Data from the Action Study revealed that employers are less likely to agree that obesity is a disease and are therefore reluctant to provide coverage. They cite concern about the cost of premiums and medical claims (52%) and the lack of data about their return on investment, treatment efficacy, and long-term benefits [2].

Although coordinated efforts are being made by professional organizations, healthcare organizations, industry partners, and other stakeholders to encourage insurers to cover obesity treatment, coverage is still limited.

4.3 Patient Barriers

Patients have their own set of barriers, which add more bricks to the wall. Their barriers include a lack of knowledge about obesity and its treatment, fear of being judged and blamed, fear of being given simplistic solutions, internalized weight bias, an uncomfortable healthcare environment, and a preference for clinicians to bring up the topic.

4.3.1 Lack of Knowledge

Lack of knowledge about weight and obesity is also common among people with obesity. However, it manifests differently than it does for clinicians. Unlike clinicians, many people with obesity do not recognize that obesity is a disease [2]. Even when they do, they don't recognize the risks to their health and life expectancy. They are also far less likely to understand the chronicity of obesity and believe that if they find the right diet, they can solve it and move on. While people with obesity are aware that they carry excess weight, they don't recognize that they have obesity. There is a perception that having obesity refers only to those who would be classified as having super-obesity, which is a BMI $\geq$ 50 kg/m^2 [2] or super-super obesity, which is a BMI $\geq$ 60 kg/m^2.

4.3.2 Belief that It's Their Responsibility

According to the Action Study, 82% of people with obesity believe that it is their sole responsibility to manage their weight [2]. If they do recognize it as a disease, they don't see it as a chronic condition, and therefore don't consider that they need assistance to manage it as they would for other chronic conditions. Even when patients recognize that their weight poses health risks and are actively engaged in efforts to lose weight, many do not consult with a healthcare provider for guidance with the process [25]. Instead, they seek answers from other sources, believing that they will find a solution and will lose their excess weight once and for all. Many have the perception that they know what they need to do to lose weight and therefore don't need the guidance of a healthcare professional [2].

Many are not aware that comprehensive, evidence-based treatment modalities such as specialized nutritional counseling, behavioral counseling, and FDA approved medications are available. While they may be aware of the benefits of bariatric surgery and procedures, they are not aware of the criteria for surgery and may believe that it is not an option for them when it may in fact be one. Very few are aware that there are primary care or specialty care clinicians who are knowledgeable about obesity and can treat or refer them to appropriate care. Even fewer know that there are clinicians who specialize in non-surgical obesity management or that the field of obesity medicine exists.

4.3.3 Fear of Being Judged and Blamed

As we learned in Chap. 2, people with obesity frequently experience weight bias and have likely been repeatedly stigmatized in healthcare settings. These experiences leave an indelible mark and influence patients' willingness to broach the topic with a healthcare professional. Many patients who have sought the help of their clinicians have been told that they are to blame for their weight gain and/or their failure to lose or maintain their weight loss. Those who have followed previous weight loss recommendations diligently and haven't lost weight have been blamed for their failure to lose. Unlike other conditions for which clinicians do not blame patients for failure to respond to the treatment regimen, such as chemotherapy for cancer or antimicrobial therapy for infections, clinicians are more likely to blame patients for failed obesity treatment than to blame the disease itself or the efficacy of the treatment.

Independent of past experiences with clinicians, patients often feel embarrassed about their weight and blame themselves for their condition, which reduces the likelihood that they will seek the assistance of their clinician to manage weight or initiate a weight-related conversation [26, 27].

4.3.4 Fear of Being Given Simplistic Solutions

Many people with obesity have made numerous attempts with little to no success. Those who have been successful have struggled to maintain their lifestyle behaviors on their own. For those who had success, metabolic adaptation has contributed to weight regain. Despite continuing the same consistent eating and exercise habits that resulted in weight loss, they have regained weight, leaving them discouraged and with the sense that further effort is futile. Because the body responds to weight loss with an increase in hunger hormones and a decrease in satiety hormones, it may become even more challenging to manage eating and limit the quantity and type of food to what was previously satisfying. Without knowledge of this physiologic reality, many see their difficulty with hunger, lack of satiety, and regain as their fault.

Because many clinicians don't know about the importance of assessing patients' own knowledge and experience by inquiring about past weight loss attempts and strategies that have been effective, they may offer suggestions such as "Eat less and move more," or "It's a simple equation: calories in versus calories out." Comments of this nature can feel completely unhelpful and potentially insulting to people who have invested considerable effort to manage their weight over the years and have found it to be far more difficult and complex than what the clinician is suggesting. This can also be the case for those who have recently embarked on the process, particularly if their efforts have not resulted in weight loss. When patients share these frustrations and the clinician responds with a comment such as, "You just need to try harder," it invalidates the effort they have expended, leaving patients feeling not only unseen, but without effective options for managing their weight. These experiences further reinforce the belief that clinicians don't have effective strategies to offer and many patients don't see the value of inquiring again.

4.3.5 Internalized Bias and Stigma

Internalization of weight bias and stigma is common among people with obesity, leading them to believe that the fault lies within themselves. As was reviewed in Chap. 2, internalized stigma has numerous negative effects on both physical and psychological health. As a result of internalized bias, patients with weight issues may not believe that they are deserving of their clinicians' attention and kindness in general, never mind if it is in regard to their weight. If they have absorbed society's narrative, they may feel they have caused their own problem and that they have "nobody to blame" but themselves. Given their previous struggles with weight loss and maintaining their loss, they may believe that asking for their clinicians' time for a discussion about their weight would be a waste of the clinicians' time. People who have internalized the entrenched societal bias and stigma about weight may reserve their harshest criticisms for themselves and believe that they are completely unworthy of any assistance whatsoever.

4.3.6   Uncomfortable Healthcare Environment

Patients commonly cite an uncomfortable healthcare environment as a reason to avoid healthcare settings altogether and as another reason not to bring up the topic of weight [28]. By the time the clinician sees a patient, that patient may have spent time in a waiting room that didn't have chairs that were large enough, may have been weighed in the hallway while other patients and staff members were nearby, and may now be squeezed into a too-small chair in the consultation room. Prior to the clinician entering the room, the patient may have experienced further discomfort when the blood pressure cuff was not of an adequate size and the medical assistant had to go searching for a "larger" one or overheard the receptionist make a snide comment about the patient's weight to a co-worker. These experiences are humiliating and do not elicit trust that a discussion about weight with the clinician will be any more comfortable than the experiences that preceded it.

4.3.7   Patients Want Clinicians to Initiate Discussions

Another reason that patients don't raise the topic is that they are looking to their clinicians to do so [29]. They see it as their clinicians' responsibility to address weight and health, so long as it's done in a sensitive and respectful manner [30]. The preference for clinician initiation may vary based on previous experiences with that particular clinician, other clinicians, and the healthcare environment, as well as other factors such as differences between clinicians' and patients' race, sex, gender, education level, and socio-economic status. Because of the inherent disparities in these factors, some patients may already feel at a significant disadvantage in the relationship, even if the clinician is sensitive and respectful. For example, an indigenous woman who has suffered abuse and is experiencing poverty may not want a white male clinician to initiate a discussion about weight based on the numerous disparities she routinely experiences, whereas a white female with a college degree might be looking to her white female clinician to bring up the topic. None of this means that the clinician can't or shouldn't bring up the topic; it is discussed to illustrate that not all patients are looking to the clinician to open the dialogue.

4.4   Dismantling the Wall and Paving a New Path

Now that we have a better understanding of the numerous barriers that patients and clinicians face, let's turn our attention to how we can remove as many bricks as possible and use them to pave a new path—one that leads to better health for people with obesity and a more rewarding experience for clinicians.

4.5   Dismantling Clinician Barriers

4.5.1   Education

The most powerful strategy for removing clinician barriers is clinician education. It has the power to remove several of the bricks from the wall, including lack of knowledge, low professional self-efficacy, low prioritization of obesity, lack of obesity-specific communication strategies, fear of making patients uncomfortable, credibility concerns, and to some degree, lack of time. Clinician education needs to occur on several levels, beginning in undergraduate and graduate programs, extending into internships and residencies, and finally into continuing education. Clinician education, particularly in undergraduate and undergraduate programs, is contingent upon faculty development in obesity management and effective obesity-specific communication strategies. Faculty includes those in academic institutions as well as clinical preceptors and others who participate in the education of clinicians-in-training.

4.5.2   Undergraduate and Graduate Education

When obesity education is included in undergraduate and graduate curricula, improved outcomes are seen [7]. In one intervention, nurse practitioner students completed a seven-module course on obesity management in primary care which included instruction on the etiology, pathophysiology, evaluation, comprehensive lifestyle interventions, pharmacology, bariatric surgery, and strategies for effective implementation. After completing the course, participants reported a significant improvement in their knowledge and comfort level with managing patients with obesity [31].

Nurse practitioner students want their curriculum to not only provide obesity education, but to provide instruction on how to initiate a discussion about weight [32]. This is consistent with other clinicians-in-training who recognize the need for obesity education in their curriculum.

4.5.3 Continuing Education

As is the case in undergraduate and graduate programs, obesity education has been shown to improve clinicians' understanding and management of obesity, as well as their professional skills and attitudes [4]. Given the prevalence of obesity, more clinicians are seeing the effects of obesity-related complications and the need to address the root cause. They recognize the need for obesity education and guidance on how to initiate and continue effective conversations about weight [3, 24].

4.5.4 Lack of Time

This is a brick that can only be partially removed. Full removal would require systemic change in the healthcare system and society. However, clinicians can address this barrier by learning how to utilize time-efficient communication strategies in which they open the conversation and schedule obesity-specific follow-up to further discuss weight and obesity treatment. Strategies for how to accomplish this will be discussed in Chaps. 6 and 7. Based on their healthcare setting and other limitations, clinicians may need to settle for shorter, less frequent appointments than is optimal, and may need to rely on referrals to other clinicians and community resources in order to provide appropriate treatment.

4.5.5 Reimbursement

Reimbursement is another heavy brick that is not easily dislodged. Insurers, employers, and government health plans in the United States hold the keys to improved reimbursement. Clinicians must work within the system to find creative ways to receive reimbursement for the time that they spend discussing weight and arranging or providing care. Knowledge of billing and coding is vital to maximizing and securing appropriate reimbursement. While this topic in an important one, it is beyond the scope of this book.

4.6 Dismantling Patient Barriers

Much of the capacity for dismantling patient barriers lies in the hands of clinicians. The education that removes clinician barriers removes patient barriers as well.

By understanding the barriers their patients face and taking targeted action, clinicians can remove the bricks of lack of knowledge about obesity, patients' belief that weight management is their responsibility, fear of being judged and blamed, fear of being given simplistic solutions, internalized bias, an uncomfortable healthcare environment, and patients' desire for clinicians to open the conversation. While clinicians do not have control over how patients respond to their efforts, they have the power to make changes in their interactions with patients and invite them to join them in creating a collaborative relationship, as well as ensuring that the healthcare environment is comfortable and accommodating. In situations where a clinician's power is limited, steady advocacy for best practices will likely bring about the desired changes with time.

4.7 Paving a New Path

Clinicians, educators, and healthcare organizations have the opportunity to re-use the bricks that once served as barriers to pave a new path. This is no small undertaking and will require the cooperation of everyone on the healthcare team, healthcare leaders, as well as policymakers, academic institutions, employers, insurers, and the public. Yes, it will take sea change, but it is possible, and frankly necessary, if we hope to improve the trajectory of the public health crisis that obesity presents around the globe.

Because clinician education is so vital to paving a new path, clinicians must take personal responsibility for educating themselves through whatever means are available to them. They can investigate the educational opportunities available in their professional and healthcare organizations, as well as local, state, and national conferences, including those that focus on obesity education. These offerings may be live in-person or virtual events; some may be available as live webinars or on-demand educational modules that can be accessed online at a time that is convenient. If adequate obesity education is not available, clinicians can request it and insist that it is offered. Requests can be communicated when completing surveys and conference evaluations or by directly contacting the organizations. See Table 4.1 for resources for further obesity education.

Professional and healthcare organizations can commit to providing and expanding options for obesity education for their clinician members and employees, including presentations at conferences, and hosting workshops, bootcamps, and online modules, as well as expanding the education to the entire healthcare team.

Educators can take responsibility for educating themselves and their colleagues and consulting with their program directors and fellow faculty members to develop plans to include and/or expand obesity education in the curriculum. This education

Table 4.1 Obesity education resources

Name of organization	Link
Obesity Medicine Association	https://obesitymedicine.org/
The Obesity Society	https://www.obesity.org/
Obesity Action Coalition	https://www.obesityaction.org/
STOP Obesity Alliance	https://stop.publichealth.gwu.edu/
The Rudd Center for Food Policy and Obesity	http://www.uconnruddcenter.org/
Obesity Canada	https://obesitycanada.ca/
World Obesity Federation	https://www.worldobesity.org/
The European Association for the Study of Obesity	https://easo.org/

can be extended to clinical preceptors as well. Chapter 3 provides information and resources for educators who want to incorporate the obesity education core competencies and benchmarks into the curriculum.

Clinicians-in training can ask instructors and program directors to add obesity education to the curriculum. They can also ask their clinical preceptors to incorporate obesity education and management opportunities into their clinical experiences. Another option is to seek obesity education from continuing education venues. Many professional organizations offer discounted rates for continuing education to clinicians-in-training.

4.8 Summary

Clinicians and patients face numerous barriers to productive conversations about weight. Many clinicians do not receive adequate education about evidence-based obesity treatment and lack confidence in their ability to effectively intervene. They also face the barriers of inadequate time, poor reimbursement, a biased healthcare system, and a fear of making patients uncomfortable. Patients also lack knowledge about obesity. Many have had negative experiences with clinicians and healthcare environments and may also believe that managing their weight is their responsibility. These barriers can be dismantled through education, the utilization of time-efficient communication strategies, and attention to the healthcare environment.

References

1. Roberts JL, Standage RP, Olaoye I, Smith LF. Overcoming barriers to weight loss practice guidelines in primary care. J Nurse Pract. 2015;11(5):544–50.
2. Kaplan LM, Golden A, Jinnett K, Kolotkin RL, Kyle TK, Look M, et al. Perceptions of barriers to effective obesity care: results from the National ACTION Study. Obesity (Silver Spring). 2018;26(1):61–9.

3. Glenister KM, Malatzky CA, Wright J. Barriers to effective conversations regarding over-weight and obesity in regional Victoria. Aust Fam Physician. 2017;46(10):769–73.
4. Sanchez-Ramirez DC, Long H, Mowat S, Hein C. Obesity education for front-line healthcare providers. BMC Med Educ. 2018;18(1):278.
5. Turner M, Jannah N, Kahan S, Gallagher C, Dietz W. Current knowledge of obesity treatment guidelines by health care professionals. Obesity (Silver Spring). 2018;26(4):665–71.
6. Srivastava G, Johnson ED, Earle RL, Kadambi N, Pazin DE, Kaplan LM. Underdocumentation of obesity by medical residents highlights challenges to effective obesity care. Obesity (Silver Spring). 2018;26(8):1277–84.
7. Mastrocola MR, Roque SS, Benning LV, Stanford FC. Obesity education in medical schools, residencies, and fellowships throughout the world: a systematic review. Int J Obes. 2020;44(2):269–79.
8. Butsch WS, Kushner RF, Alford S, Smolarz BG. Low priority of obesity education leads to lack of medical students' preparedness to effectively treat patients with obesity: results from the U.S. medical school obesity education curriculum benchmark study. BMC Med Educ. 2020;20(1):23.
9. Bleich SN, Bandara S, Bennett WL, Cooper LA, Gudzune KA. U.S. health professionals' views on obesity care, training, and self-efficacy. Am J Prev Med. 2015;48(4):411–8.
10. Jay M, Gillespie C, Ark T, Richter R, McMacken M, Zabar S, et al. Do internists, pediatricians, and psychiatrists feel competent in obesity care?: using a needs assessment to drive curriculum design. J Gen Intern Med. 2008;23(7):1066–70.
11. Puhl RM, Heuer CA. The stigma of obesity: a review and update. Obesity (Silver Spring). 2009;17(5):941–64.
12. Sturgiss E, Haesler E, Elmitt N, van Weel C, Douglas K. Increasing general practitioners' confidence and self-efficacy in managing obesity: a mixed methods study. BMJ Open. 2017;7(1):e014314.
13. Smith S, Seeholzer EL, Gullett H, Jackson B, Antognoli E, Krejci SA, et al. Primary care residents' knowledge, attitudes, self-efficacy, and perceived professional norms regarding obesity, nutrition, and physical activity counseling. J Grad Med Educ. 2015;7(3):388–94.
14. Hauff C, Fruh SM, Sims BM, Williams SG, Herf C, Golden A, et al. Nurse practitioner students' observations of preceptor engagement in obesity management and weight bias: a mixed-methods approach. J Am Assoc Nurse Pract. 2020;32(7):520–9.
15. Petrin C, Kahan S, Turner M, Gallagher C, Dietz WH. Current attitudes and practices of obesity counselling by health care providers. Obes Res Clin Pract. 2017;11(3):352–9.
16. Reto CS. Psychological aspects of delivering nursing care to the bariatric patient. Crit Care Nurs Q. 2003;26(2):139–49.
17. Ahmed SM, Lemkau JP, Birt SL. Toward sensitive treatment of obese patients. Fam Pract Manag. 2002;9(1):25–8.
18. Keyworth C, Peters S, Chisholm A, Hart J. Nursing students' perceptions of obesity and behaviour change: implications for undergraduate nurse education. Nurse Educ Today. 2013;33(5):481–5.
19. Phelan SM, Dovidio JF, Puhl RM, Burgess DJ, Nelson DB, Yeazel MW, et al. Implicit and explicit weight bias in a national sample of 4732 medical students: the medical student CHANGES study. Obesity (Silver Spring). 2014;22(4):1201–8.
20. Bleich SN, Bennett WL, Gudzune KA, Cooper LA. Impact of physician BMI on obesity care and beliefs. Obesity (Silver Spring). 2012;20(5):999–1005.
21. Bleich SN, Gudzune KA, Bennett WL, Jarlenski MP, Cooper LA. How does physician BMI impact patient trust and perceived stigma? Prev Med. 2013;57(2):120–4.
22. Bleich SN, Bandara S, Bennett WL, Cooper LA, Gudzune KA. Impact of non-physician health professionals' BMI on obesity care and beliefs. Obesity (Silver Spring). 2014;22(12):2476–80.
23. Hague AL, White AA. Web-based intervention for changing attitudes of obesity among current and future teachers. J Nutr Educ Behav. 2005;37(2):58–66.

24. Phillips K, Wood F, Kinnersley P. Tackling obesity: the challenge of obesity management for practice nurses in primary care. Fam Pract. 2014;31(1):51–9.
25. Stokes A, Collins JM, Grant BF, Hsiao CW, Johnston SS, Ammann EM, et al. Prevalence and determinants of engagement with obesity care in the United States. Obesity (Silver Spring). 2018;26(5):814–8.
26. Malterud K, Ulriksen K. Obesity in general practice: a focus group study on patient experiences. Scand J Prim Health Care. 2010;28(4):205–10.
27. Mensinger JL, Tylka TL, Calamari ME. Mechanisms underlying weight status and healthcare avoidance in women: a study of weight stigma, body-related shame and guilt, and healthcare stress. Body Image. 2018;25:139–47.
28. Merrill E, Grassley J. Women's stories of their experiences as overweight patients. J Adv Nurs. 2008;64(2):139–46.
29. Look M, Kolotkin RL, Dhurandhar NV, Nadglowski J, Stevenin B, Golden A. Implications of differing attitudes and experiences between providers and persons with obesity: results of the national ACTION study. Postgrad Med. 2019;131(5):357–65.
30. Koball AM, Mueller PS, Craner J, Clark MM, Nanda S, Kebede EB, et al. Crucial conversations about weight management with healthcare providers: patients' perspectives and experiences. Eat Weight Disord. 2018;23(1):87–94.
31. Fruh SM, Golden A, Graves RJ, Minchew LA, Platt TH, Hall HR, et al. Competency in obesity management: an educational intervention study with nurse practitioner students. J Am Assoc Nurse Pract. 2019;31(12):734–40.
32. Fruh SM, Golden A, Graves RJ, Hall HR, Minchew LA, Williams S. Advanced practice nursing student knowledge in obesity management: a mixed methods research study. Nurse Educ Today. 2019;77:59–64.

Chapter 5
Creating an Environment for Effective Conversation

5.1 Introduction

The clinical environment sets the stage for effective conversations. When the environment is weight inclusive and welcoming, patients are more likely to have a positive experience. When it is not, it is another experience in which patients with obesity encounter weight bias in healthcare settings. Negative experiences caused by the clinical environment inflict harm and increase the likelihood that patients won't return for follow-up care. The physical environment and the emotional experiences patients have need to be safe, accessible, accommodating, comfortable, welcoming, and non-shaming. This requires attention to both the built environment and the manner in which all members of the healthcare team communicate with patients with obesity. If either experience is uncomfortable, it is more likely that a patient will have an overall negative experience. This chapter provides guidance on how to ensure that clinical spaces and equipment are size inclusive and that all office and clinical support staff know how to interact with patients in a sensitive, respectful manner.

5.2 Creating a Positive Physical Environment

When entering healthcare settings, patients with obesity may find themselves in an environment that requires them to navigate numerous physical obstacles such as furniture and equipment that do not safely or comfortably accommodate their bodies.

Women report themes of "struggling to fit in" when entering a healthcare setting, citing the need to squeeze into inadequate seating, gowns that are not large enough, paper drapes that are too small, and inadequately sized blood pressure cuffs and speculums [1]. Because concerns about inadequate furniture and equipment prevent

© Springer Nature Switzerland AG 2021
S. Christensen, *A Clinician's Guide to Discussing Obesity with Patients*,
https://doi.org/10.1007/978-3-030-69311-4_5

patients from visiting their clinicians [2], it is of high importance that healthcare environments have appropriately sized furniture and equipment.

The first obstacle may appear as soon as patients open the waiting room door. If the pathway between the door and the reception desk is not wide enough due to furniture placement and/or is impeded by other patients exiting the clinic, their first seconds in the clinic are uncomfortable both physically and emotionally. The next obstacle might be encountering chairs in the waiting room and clinical areas that are not large enough or sturdy enough, which may also be the case for exam tables and other furniture upon which they will stand, sit, or lie. Doorways and hallways may also be too narrow, creating further obstacles. For these reasons, care and forethought should be given to every aspect of the physical encounter from the moment of the patient's entry until the final exit.

In one study of nurse practitioner students, students reported inappropriate equipment and inadequate privacy for patients with obesity in their clinical rotations [3]. Students noted the lack of adequately sized gowns for patient exams and the use of paper gowns that did not adequately cover the patients as they waited for their clinicians and during the visit and examination. They further noted that when clinical staff needed to leave the room to locate adequately sized equipment, it increased the risk of patients feeling self-conscious.

These students also reported weighing procedures that lacked privacy or sensitivity or that took place in areas that inadequately accommodated patients with obesity. They encountered scales in open areas or in wall nooks that were too narrow, which required them to be pulled out of the nook in order for the patient to be weighed. Students noted that when this was done in front of a patient it caused unnecessary embarrassment [3]. These students recalled hearing the medical assistant or nurse calling out the patient's weight when the scale was in an open area [3]. Some students heard nurses, clinical staff, and receptionists make derogatory comments about patients, at times within earshot of those patients.

5.2.1 Furniture

Chairs and sofas in the waiting area, exam rooms, procedure rooms, and other areas in which patients will sit should be large enough, sturdy enough, and firm enough to accommodate persons who weigh up to 600 pounds. If possible, it is advisable to have a selection of chair widths, particularly in waiting areas, so that patients can select the chair width that is most comfortable and appropriate for them. While it is important to provide furniture that can accommodate all body sizes, some patients feel self-conscious if the only chair available to them is substantially larger than they require. Sofas and love seats provide further options for those who feel self-conscious about sitting in a larger chair than is needed, with the added benefit of accommodating those with super obesity and super-super obesity. It is optimal to have some chairs with arms and some without. Armless chairs accommodate larger bodies without the risk of the patient becoming stuck between the armrests.

However, those with orthopedic concerns that affect the hips and lower limbs find that arms are useful, and in some cases necessary, when sitting down and rising from a chair. All seating should have firm cushions, as they are easier for patients to sit in and arise from. If the cushion is too soft or too low, it can cause physical pain when patients sit down and stand up, or require them to ask for assistance, potentially causing embarrassment.

In order to prevent tipping, exam tables should be wide and sturdy with a capacity of up to 600 pounds [4]. This is also true for tables in procedure rooms and operating rooms. It is important to verify in advance that a procedure table has the capacity for the person scheduled, as it can be distressing for a patient to arrive for a procedure and be told that it can't be done due to the inadequate weight capacity or width of the table. Sturdy step stools with handles that have an adequate weight capacity should be available for patients to climb onto the exam or procedure table [4].

All furniture should be placed in a manner that provides easy access and a path that is wide enough to accommodate them as they move from one area to another and doesn't put them in awkward situations when encountering staff or other patients in hallways. Toilets should be floor mounted and able to sustain higher weights. Split toilet seats are advisable [4].

5.2.2   Scales

One of the most vital pieces of equipment is the scale. When healthcare settings do not have scales that accommodate people with higher weights, it can create an exquisitely uncomfortable experience for them. Unfortunately, far too many people with super obesity can recount painful experiences of stepping on a scale and being told that they weigh more than the scale can read. Although it rarely happens anymore, some have been sent to junkyards [5] or livestock scales to get an accurate weight reading. Even when the clinical staff communicates with tenderness and compassion, the experience is likely to feel humiliating and shaming. This is why it is vital to have at least one scale that can accommodate weights greater than 500 pounds. If that is not possible, it is advisable to make arrangements in advance to have patients weighed on a scale that has adequate capacity.

Scales should be placed in private areas where only the patient and person measuring the weight can see the reading. They should not be placed in hallways, near the desks of clinic staff, or in other public areas. As is the case for furniture, the pathway to and from the scale should be of an adequate width with no obstacles. The platform of the scale should be placed far enough from the wall so that there is room between the person and the wall. Because abdominal girth can make it difficult to see the platform onto which they are stepping, there should be a sturdy handle or surface that the patient can use for balance and stability when getting on and off the scale.

5.2.3   *Equipment*

All equipment that is used during the patient encounter should have the capacity to measure accurately and prevent any physical or emotional discomfort for the patient. The costs of not having appropriate-sized equipment are great. Not only is the clinical staff unable to obtain accurate information about the health status of their patients, inappropriately sized equipment can cause unnecessary physical pain for patients and create situations that cause embarrassment and generate shame. If failure to have the correct equipment necessitates an appointment to be rescheduled, patients experience unnecessary inconvenience. Given that negative experiences contribute to patients with obesity canceling appointments or failing to return for follow-up, attention to equipment improves the likelihood that patients will have a positive experience and return in the future.

Large and thigh-sized blood pressure cuffs should be readily available and used for those with an upper arm circumference greater than 34 cm. If the cuff is too small, the reading will not be accurate. Additionally, there is a possibility that the cuff will pop off when it is being inflated, creating an embarrassing situation for the patient. Ideally, adequately sized blood pressure cuffs should be available in every room. Tape measures that are used for measuring waist circumference should be at least 72 inches. Extra-large gowns and drapes should also be available. When gowns or drapes do not adequately cover a patient, it can be both physically and emotionally uncomfortable. When collecting specimens, it is advisable to have extra-long needles for blood draws, large vaginal speculums, and urine specimen collectors that have a handle [4]. All equipment should be gathered in advance so that the clinical staff doesn't have to go searching for it in the middle of the procedure, potentially creating uncomfortable situations for patients. When proper sized equipment isn't available—particularly vaginal speculums—clinicians are less likely to perform procedures such as pelvic exams, which contributes to less screening for women with obesity [6].

Table 5.1 provides a list of the appropriate furniture and equipment that are needed to safely and comfortably accommodate patients with obesity.

Table 5.1 Safe, comfortable, accommodating furniture and equipment

Furniture with capacity to support 600 pounds	Equipment
Firm chairs, some with arms, some without	Scales with a capacity of 600 pounds with handlebars
Firm sofas	Large and thigh sized blood pressure cuffs (larger than 34 cm)
Wide, sturdy exam tables	Tape measures that are at least 72 inches long
Wide, sturdy procedure tables	Large patient gowns and drapes
Sturdy step stools with handlebars	Extra-long vaginal speculums
Floor mounted toilets with split seats	Extra-long needles for blood draws
	Urine specimen collectors with handles

5.3 Creating a Positive Emotional Environment

In addition to ensuring that patients are physically comfortable, attention needs to be given to making patients emotionally comfortable. From the information on the website to their first conversation with office staff to the literature in the waiting room, patients receive messages about whether or not they will have an emotionally comfortable experience. Given the negative experiences that many people with obesity have had in clinical settings, they are particularly sensitive to language and practices that suggest that they may have another unpleasant encounter. In order for patients to gain enough trust to schedule an appointment and continue the recommended follow-up, all members of the healthcare team need to be educated about the importance of positive communication and be trained in how to interact in a sensitive and respectful manner.

While the bulk of the conversations about obesity will take place between the clinician and patient, patients interact with other staff members when both scheduling and attending appointments. For this reason, all staff should be educated about how to talk to, and about, patients with obesity, including using People First Language (PFL). Although it is not necessary to educate them on the pathophysiology of obesity, it is important that they understand that obesity is a chronic disease that requires comprehensive, long-term treatment. They need to understand the prevalence of weight bias and stigma and the negative effects it has on patients' physical and psychological health so that they understand why it is vital to ensure that interactions are free of bias and stigmatization. It is the standard of care that all conversations about patients should take place behind closed doors. However, there may be times when staff members are not careful and patients or others in the clinic overhear phone calls or conversations, making it all the more important that all staff speak accurately and respectfully about both the patient and the treatment process, and are using PFL. It is vitally important that all staff avoid making hurtful comments or jokes about patients with obesity [4]. Although it may be obvious that such behavior is unacceptable, this is a point that needs to be emphasized. In a study examining the experiences that nurse practitioner students had with their preceptors in women's health outpatient settings, one student commented, "I have heard insults and stereotyping amongst the non-clinical staff/receptionists before and after seeing certain patients." [3].

The key to reducing weight bias and stigmatization is education, which is why the importance of staff education can't be overstated.

5.3.1 Clinic Websites and Literature

Prior to their first appointment, patients often review clinic websites and brochures to determine what type of experience they can expect to have, making it important to send the correct message. If there is information about obesity treatment, it is

Table 5.2 Obesity image galleries

Image gallery	Link
Obesity Action Coalition Image Gallery	https://www.obesityaction.org/get-educated/public-resources/oac-image-gallery/
U-Conn Rudd Center Image Gallery	http://www.uconnruddcenter.org/media-gallery
Obesity Canada Image Bank	https://obesitycanada.ca/resources/image-bank/
World Obesity Federation Image Bank	https://www.worldobesity.org/resources/image-bank

important that the message focuses on health, rather than weight loss. When images of patients are used in promotional materials and websites, particularly if obesity treatment is offered, images should be selected from image galleries that show people with obesity in a positive light. Table 5.2 provides information on how to access these galleries, which include a variety of images of people with obesity cooking healthy food, exercising, and interacting with friends, family, and colleagues. Images that show people with obesity eating junk food, that only show them from the back, or cut off their heads as though their bodies are too shameful to show their faces, perpetuate stigmatizing stereotypes. Although it is common, it is not advisable to show "before and after" images of patients. Given that successful treatment often results in a modest weight reduction, seeing images and hearing stories of those who have had greater loss can be discouraging and minimize the significant health benefits of a modest loss. These images emphasize weight loss rather than the health benefits of effective obesity treatment.

Waiting rooms and exam rooms often contain reading materials such as magazines, brochures, and other periodicals. This literature must be carefully selected to ensure that it promotes health and focuses on healthy behaviors, rather than dieting, thinness, beauty, glamor, and food. It sends a mixed message if the clinical staff focuses on health, but the environment glamorizes unattainable body and beauty images or promotes unhealthy food.

5.3.2   Office Staff

Because the first encounter patients have is often with the front desk staff, it is just as important that they have a framework for conversations as it is for the clinical support staff and clinicians. Whether they are interacting with patients, families, internal clinic staff, external offices and agencies, or insurance companies, they should be well-versed in using phrases such as *the woman with obesity* or *the man affected by obesity* and refrain from using the terms *obese*, *morbidly obese*, *fat*, and other words and phrases that are derogatory. When personnel such as the referral coordinator or insurance biller interact with patients, families, external clinicians and their staff, agencies, and insurers, their use of PFL models respectful, informed communication about the disease of obesity and those affected by it in a manner that will shift thinking away from stigmatization towards recognizing obesity as a treatable health condition.

5.3.3 Clinical Staff

The clinical staff includes nurses, social workers, medical assistants, technicians, nutritionists, phlebotomists, and other professionals and assistants. All interact with patients and should understand the importance of sensitive, respectful language, as well as practices that protect the privacy and dignity of the patient.

It is ideal if all readings, including weight, vital signs, and waist circumference are done in a private area. Prior to bringing a patient into the clinical area, the medical assistant should assemble all equipment in advance so that the patient will have a smooth experience. Not doing so could result in a situation that causes discomfort or embarrassment. An example of such a situation is wrapping the wrong sized blood pressure cuff around a patient's arm only to discover that it is too small and a larger one needs to be located. If the staff member adds a comment such as, "This cuff is too small for you," or worse yet, "Your arm is too big for this cuff, I'll have to go find the extra-large one," the patient is likely to feel judged and embarrassed. Although these may seem like innocuous comments, patients are very sensitive to any language that conveys negativity about their body size. If a staff member finds that the cuff is too small, it is better to say something such as, "I'm sorry, I didn't use the correct cuff. I will go locate the correct one." The same is true for having a long vaginal speculum in the room prior to a pelvic exam, large gowns and drapes in the room, and extra-long needles readily available for blood draws.

Patients should be weighed in a private area in which the reading cannot be seen by others. Before patients step on the scale it is advisable to ask if they want to know their weight or not. If they do not, they can stand on the scale facing away from the readout so that they don't have to see it. If they want to know, they can face the display and see it for themselves. Regardless of whether the patient sees the weight or not, it should be written in the chart without comment. Evaluative comments such as "That's good," or "You are doing great," even if they are intended to encourage, can be uncomfortable for the patient and potentially set them up for feeling judged or that they have disappointed the staff member if there is no weight loss or there is a gain at a future weighing. Although it is obvious, comments about weight gain such as, "You've gained weight," or "Your weight is up," could be construed as criticism. If the patient wants to know, it is fine to provide the weight. However, conversations about the implications of the reading on the scale or vital signs are best left for the clinician and the patient.

5.3.4 Training Modules and Procedures

All new clinical and office staff should receive training about the manner in which they should discuss obesity and weight-related topics with patients, family, and other members of the clinical team. It is important for them to understand the consequences of their actions and how the manner in which they approach patients can have a positive or negative impact on their health and well-being. Without an awareness of the harm that can be done, it may be difficult for staff to understand the importance of their actions.

Annual training should be conducted to ensure that all staff are up to date on the best practices for ensuring a positive physical and emotional environment for patients with obesity. These trainings should include reminders, and ideally opportunities, to self-reflect on their biases in order to increase rapport with their patients with obesity [3].

5.4 Clinical Scenarios

The following scenarios provide examples of staff-patient interactions that are insensitive or shaming. Each provides a more appropriate interaction that is sensitive and respectful. This will guide you in teaching best practices to all staff members.

Scenario 1
A medical assistant is weighing a female patient prior to an appointment with the clinician.
   Medical assistant: "It's 217.4 pounds. You've gained weight. Are you having trouble with your diet?"
   Appropriate Interaction
   Prior to weighing the patient, the medical assistant asked for the patient's preference.
   Medical assistant: "Would you like to know your weight today?"
   Patient: "Yes."
   Medical Assistant: "It's 217.4 pounds."

5.4.1 Discussion

In the first interaction, the medical assistant did not ask the patient if she wanted to know her weight prior to telling her, which did not show respect. The comment, "You've gained weight," has the potential to sound judgmental to the patient. The additional comment, "Are you having trouble with your diet?" is stigmatizing, as it implies that the weight gain is the result of overeating. Additionally, this question is outside of the medical assistant's scope of practice.

In the appropriate interaction, the medical assistant asked the patient's preference and appropriately provided the weight without additional comments.

Scenario 2

The medical assistant is in the exam room taking the patient's blood pressure. He wraps the blood pressure cuff on the patient's arm and realizes it isn't large enough for the patient's arm.

Medical assistant: "This cuff is too small. You need a bigger one."

He then opens the exam room door and yells to a colleague down the hall, "Hey can you get the large thigh cuff and bring it to room 3. Thanks!"

Appropriate Interaction

Prior to bringing the patient to the exam room, the medical assistant checks to ensure that all blood pressure cuff sizes are available in the room. No comments are made about the size of the cuff.

5.4.2 Discussion

In the first example, the medical assistant did not consider the patient's comfort by locating the correct sized cuff prior to taking the blood pressure. The comments "This cuff is too small," and "You need a bigger one," are insensitive to the patient and could be interpreted as a judgement about the patient's body size. Additional pain and embarrassment were caused when the medical assistant yelled the need for a bigger cuff down the hall.

In the appropriate interaction, the medical assistant showed sensitivity by gathering the appropriate-sized cuff prior to bringing the patient to the room. If the patient's size had been unknown to the medical assistant prior to bringing the patient to the room, he should locate the cuff without comment.

Scenario 3

A clinic scheduler is on the phone with a patient who needs to schedule an appointment.

Patient: "I recently had bariatric surgery and need to come in for a rash I've had on my abdomen since the surgery."

Scheduler: "Since you are obese, we'll need to schedule you in the big room and allow extra time for the medical assistant to weigh you and take your vital signs."

This conversation is overheard by those in the waiting room.

Appropriate Interaction
"Yes, we can see you. Your appointment will take 20 min." The scheduler assigned the patient to the room that has furniture and equipment that can accommodate the patient. A note was made on the schedule to notify the medical assistant to check the room prior to rooming the patient to ensure that all necessary equipment is available.

5.4.3 Discussion

In the first interaction, the scheduler used derogatory language (obese) when speaking to the patient, which is not consistent with PFL. This is not only hurtful to the patient, it perpetuates the use of derogatory language, particularly because it could be overheard by others in the clinic. Further damage was caused when the scheduler referred to the "big" room and voiced the need for "extra time" due to the patient's size, which were heard by both the patient and others in the clinic. These comments were shaming to both the patient and anyone else with weight issues who may have overheard them.

In the appropriate interaction, the scheduler correctly identified that this patient needs to be seen in a room with the appropriate-sized furniture and equipment, proactively noted it on the schedule, and alerted the medical assistant in advance, all without commenting on it to the patient. These actions demonstrate sensitivity and respect and pave the way for a smooth, non-shaming experience for the patient.

Scenario 4
A patient approaches the reception desk to check in for an appointment with her PCP who is managing her obesity. There are other patients sitting in the waiting room.
    Receptionist: "Hi Sarah, are you here for your weight loss appointment?"
    Alternative Interaction
    Receptionist: "Hi Sarah, thanks for checking in. I'll let them know you are here."

5.4.4 Discussion

In the first example, the receptionist did not protect the patient's privacy. Although she is personable and friendly, she disclosed the patient's protected healthcare to the other patients in the waiting room. This is not only a breach of confidentiality; it has the potential to hurt and embarrass the patient.

In the appropriate interaction the receptionist was personable and friendly, while protecting the patient's privacy.

Scenario 5

A patient is meeting with the insurance coordinator to discuss coverage for bariatric surgery.

Insurance coordinator: "It looks like your insurance doesn't cover bariatric surgery."

Patient: "That's very disappointing. I really need some help with my weight, and this is what my nurse practitioner recommended."

Insurance Coordinator: "My sister did Weight Watchers and she lost over 70 pounds. She said it wasn't that hard. Maybe you should try it too."

Alternative Interaction

Insurance coordinator: "It looks like your insurance doesn't cover bariatric surgery."

Patient: "That's very disappointing. I really need some help with my weight, and this is what my nurse practitioner recommended."

Insurance Coordinator: "I'm sorry that you don't have coverage. Would you like me to ask the scheduler to make you an appointment with your nurse practitioner to discuss other treatment options?"

5.4.5 Discussion

In the first interaction the scheduler stepped out of her role of insurance coordinator and into that of a clinician. It is inappropriate for the coordinator to suggest treatment options. The suggestion that losing 70 pounds "wasn't that hard" is not consistent with the science of obesity treatment. Furthermore, it sets the patient up to feel like a failure if similar results are not achieved or if there have been previous unsuccessful efforts.

In the alternative interaction the coordinator showed empathy and appropriately directed the patient back to the clinician for further discussion on treatment options.

5.5 Summary

Conversations about obesity are most effective when they take place in a healthcare setting that is weight inclusive and welcoming. This is accomplished by creating a positive physical and emotional environment. Attention must be given to ensure that the built environment and all furniture and equipment are safe and can accommodate patients with obesity. All staff need to be educated about how to communicate with sensitivity and respect. Negative experiences with either the physical or emotional environment cause harm to patients and decrease the likelihood that they will access healthcare in the future.

References

1. Merrill E, Grassley J. Women's stories of their experiences as overweight patients. J Adv Nurs. 2008;64(2):139–46.
2. Mensinger JL, Tylka TL, Calamari ME. Mechanisms underlying weight status and healthcare avoidance in women: a study of weight stigma, body-related shame and guilt, and healthcare stress. Body Image. 2018;25:139–47.
3. Hauff C, Fruh SM, Graves RJ, Sims BM, Williams SG, Minchew LA, et al. NP student encounters with obesity bias in clinical practice. Nurse Pract. 2019;44(6):41–6.
4. Bays HE, McCarthy W, Christensen S, Tondt J, Karjoo S, Davisson L, Ng J, Golden A, Burridge K, Conroy R, Wells S, Umashanker D, Afreen S, DeJesus R, Salter D, Shah N. Obesity algorithm eBook. Obesity Medicine Association; 2020. https://obesitymedicine.org/obesity-algorithm/.
5. Bramblette S. I am not obese. I am just fat. Narrative Inquiry in Bioethics. 2014;4(2):85–8. https://doi.org/10.1353/nib.2014.0030.
6. Ferrante JM, Fyffe DC, Vega ML, Piasecki AK, Ohman-Strickland PA, Crabtree BF. Family physicians' barriers to cancer screening in extremely obese patients. Obesity (Silver Spring). 2010;18(6):1153–9.

Chapter 6
Creating a Framework for Effective Conversations

6.1 Introduction

Effective conversations about obesity and weight are the gateway to effective treatment and improved health. Despite the barriers, it is possible to structure a conversation in a manner in which the topic can be introduced in a respectful, time-efficient manner. This chapter will provide you with a framework, as well as specific techniques that can be used. It will provide guidance on how to select patients who will be receptive to your inquiries, how to broach the topic, how to structure the initial conversation so that it can take place in 5 min or less, and how to set the stage for further conversation.

6.2 Build a Partnership

A collaborative, respectful clinician-patient relationship is the scaffolding from which effective conversations take place. Regardless of a clinician's knowledge about obesity, productive conversations occur when clinicians focus on building a trusting partnership that informs and empowers. From the beginning, conscious effort must be made to counter the effects of the bias, stigmatization, and discrimination that patients have experienced in healthcare. This is accomplished through attunement to language and behaviors that may indicate prior negative experiences, and by providing a collaborative, respectful experience that is free of judgement. Through words and behaviors, you can send the message: *It's you and me against the disease.*

The attitude that you bring to the conversation is more important than the specifics of what you say. Attempting new behaviors feels awkward at first but with time and experience, skills improve. We often learn as much from our missteps as we do from our successes. Your sincere dedication to getting it right is felt by your patients.

© Springer Nature Switzerland AG 2021
S. Christensen, *A Clinician's Guide to Discussing Obesity with Patients*,
https://doi.org/10.1007/978-3-030-69311-4_6

When they know you are on their side and you make a communication error, they are likely to forgive you, stay connected, and move on. When you recognize that you have made an error or have been insensitive, set things right by apologizing and expressing your desire to maintain a positive relationship.

When patients experience genuine curiosity and compassion from their clinicians, they feel seen and accepted. With time they will internalize those qualities, resulting in a more curious mindset and the cultivation of greater self-compassion. Both are needed to establish and maintain the health behaviors that are required to successfully manage obesity. This type of interaction is in stark contrast to the all-too-common experience in which patients internalize weight bias from their healthcare providers.

6.3   Seek the Patient's Perspective

One of the most powerful strategies for building a clinician-patient partnership is for clinicians to inquire about their patients' perspective about their weight, health, and motivation. The process of inquiring about the patient's perspective with interest and sincerity is a therapeutic intervention in itself. Not only does it provide clinicians with valuable information that will guide the conversation and treatment plan, patients internalize the process and gain an improved ability for self-inquiry that allows them to get in touch with their own wisdom and answers. Your inquiries should take place in the beginning phases of a conversation about weight and be continued throughout the discussion. If you are providing obesity management care to your patient, the inquiry process is an invaluable clinical tool that should be continued throughout treatment. If you are seeing the patient for another reason while they are receiving obesity care from another clinician, your inquiries about their treatment experiences provide them with valuable support and further solidify their commitment. If your patient has dropped out of obesity care, your interest and empathy may rekindle your patient's commitment to health. In such a situation, the tools of inquiry and understanding may be just what your patient needs to reengage.

Regardless of the reason they are seeking healthcare, patients with obesity frequently receive unsolicited advice to lose weight without any inquiry as to their current or past efforts. They are rarely asked for their perspective about their weight, health, motivation, previous attempts, or if they are currently engaged in weight reduction. These experiences leave patients feeling judged and unseen, particularly in cases in which patients are actively losing weight or have lost weight in the past and are successfully maintaining their weight loss. Not only do these experiences erode the clinician-patient relationship, they may sever it completely, and contribute to people with obesity choosing to delay or avoid healthcare altogether [1]. The following scenario provides an example of this all-too-common experience.

A patient is seeing an orthopedic provider for a knee issue that is causing pain. The patient sees an obesity specialist regularly and has lost 60 pounds in the past 15 months. The patient has been riding an exercise bike for 15–30 min a day for the past 9 months and knee pain arose recently during one of those sessions. The patient has been unable to ride since that time due to the pain and has come for an evaluation by the orthopedic provider. The orthopedic provider has taken a history on the knee problem and without inquiring about the patient's weight history or physical activity history, the clinician says, "Your knee would hurt less if you lost some weight."

This clinician demonstrated bias and did not make any attempt to seek the patient's perspective or build the clinician-patient relationship. As a result, the experience felt stigmatizing and invalidating to a patient who is actively managing obesity and is regularly engaging in physical activity.

Research shows that there are discrepancies between clinicians' and patients' perceptions as to patients' motivation to manage their weight. Clinicians have an explicit belief that patients aren't motivated to lose weight [2–5], whereas patients report much higher levels of motivation [6]. These discrepancies occur because clinicians don't inquire about their patients' motivation and instead make biased assumptions, highlighting the need for clinicians to seek their patients' perspective.

Many patients have made numerous attempts to lose weight and maintain the loss and have insights about what has worked and what hasn't. They are often aware of their strengths and the places where they have encountered challenges. Inquiries about their previous attempts—what worked, what didn't, and their perspective on the factors that contributed to the outcome of those events—provide clinicians with valuable information about how to formulate a treatment plan. These inquiries also provide an opportunity for clinicians to educate their patients about the challenges of weight management and the chronic nature of obesity. All too often patients internalize the idea that they haven't tried hard enough despite all the effort they have expended. They believe that past difficulties with weight loss, maintaining consistent health behaviors, or regaining weight while consistently maintaining their health behaviors are evidence that they have done something wrong. When clinicians recognize this belief, they can remind patients that their struggles with their weight aren't as much about their efforts as they are about the physiological and environmental challenges they face. This helps patients release some of their shame and internalized bias, further strengthening the therapeutic alliance. It reinforces the concept of: *It's you and me against the disease.*

6.4   Select Appropriate Patients

As you consider opening discussions about weight with your patients, you may feel overwhelmed by the sheer number of patients who would benefit from the discussion. Because it's impossible to open the conversation with everyone, especially in the beginning, it's best to start with a few patients and build momentum. This gives you the space to practice your skills and refine your approach before expanding your reach. It is best to choose patients who you feel are most likely to be receptive, which will likely be patients with whom you already have a positive, trusting relationship.

It is advisable broach the topic during an appointment in which adequate time has been scheduled. An ideal situation is during the yearly wellness visit, when the focus is on reviewing the health history, reviewing existing health problems, addressing patient concerns, and determining which health issues could become a concern in the future so that they can be addressed before they become problematic. Other opportunities include diabetes follow-up visits and other follow-up visits that have been scheduled to manage the complications of obesity.

6.5   Guiding Concepts for Conversation

During any conversation about weight, clinicians should be guided by three concepts—focus on health, focus on the long-game, and use appropriate language.

6.5.1   Focus on Health

When initiating conversations about weight and obesity, the focus should be on health, rather than weight or appearance. Conversations—and treatment—are more effective when they are health-centric, rather than weight-centric. This requires clinicians to shift their mindset from discussing weight to supporting health. Health-centric conversations improve the chance that patients will engage in health behaviors that prevent, improve or resolve obesity-related complications, improve quality of life, and lead to successful long-term health and weight management. Patients report that when their clinicians initiate discussions with an imperative to lose weight without any mention of their health it feels like a judgement, rather than a concern about their health. As a result, patients delay care out of fear that they will receive unsolicited advice to lose weight from their clinicians [7].

Helping patients make the connection between their current concerns, symptoms, and function and their lifestyle choices, increases their motivation and focus. This strategy puts an emphasis on the here and now, rather than the elusive future. Most patients care about their health but struggle to connect today's choices to future health. Clinicians are often far more aware of potential obesity complications than their patients are. It is more difficult to connect today's choices with health outcomes in 5–10 or even 20 years, than to connect them to how it will feel to live life tomorrow.

6.5.2   Focus on the Long Game

Given the chronic nature of obesity, it is best to focus on the long game. Obesity will not be resolved in one appointment. Because it will require a series of conversations over the course of months to years, it is best to conduct each encounter in a manner that will lead to future conversations. In the case that you may only have one conversation with a particular patient, it is advisable to consider the conversations that patient may have with other clinicians in the future and focus on making it a positive experience. Successful obesity management requires all members of the healthcare team—even those who do not know or practice with the other members of the team—to accomplish what is possible and set the stage for future conversations. A positive, respectful experience makes it far more likely that patients will be receptive to discussing their weight with healthcare providers in the future. There will be times when patients are not receptive to your efforts. If that is the case, it is best to honor their wishes, end the conversation, and inform them that the door is always open for future conversations. This honors their autonomy and demonstrates respect for their wishes. It is appropriate and advisable to bring up the topic again at future encounters, when they may be more receptive. Future receptivity is based on the experience they have had with you in the past, reinforcing the importance of maintaining a positive clinician-patient partnership.

6.5.3   Use Appropriate Language

Language is a powerful tool. That's why the type of language we use when discussing weight and obesity with patients matters. Given the bias and stigma that many with obesity have experienced, particularly in healthcare, clinicians must use language that makes patients feel welcome and respected and avoid language that is stigmatizing and dehumanizing. The primary goal of any conversation is to build a collaborative, respectful clinician-patient relationship, for this will increase the likelihood that patients will continue to seek healthcare. As discussed in Chap. 2, when patients experience bias and stigma, they are far less likely to return for follow-up care and worse health outcomes are seen.

An important guiding principle is to approach patients with obesity with the same respect, compassion, and clinical mindset that you use when approaching patients with any other health condition, whether it is chronic—diabetes, hypertension, autoimmune disorders—or acute, such as infections or injuries. This mindset will keep you focused on the fact that obesity is a chronic condition and that patients need you to treat them as you would any other patient with a serious health issue. Keeping this in mind informs you about the importance of using language that is therapeutic and empowering, not stigmatizing. Non-stigmatizing language increases motivation to change behavior, particularly when the focus is on specific health behaviors as opposed to weight.

6.5.4 People-First Language

People-first language (PFL) for obesity promotes patient-centered care and should always be used when speaking to or about patients with obesity. PFL puts the person before the disease and is used by clinicians when referring to other chronic health and mental health conditions such as diabetes, depression, and autism. It is also used when referencing or speaking to people with disabilities or those who are experiencing poverty or homelessness. PFL for obesity is supported by several national and international professional associations in the U.S., Canada, and Europe, and the list is growing (Obesity Action Coalition, n.d.; Obesity Canada, n.d.). These organizations understand the importance of avoiding biased language and stand as examples of what organizations can do to support non-stigmatizing language.

PFL for obesity refrains from using labels such as *obese* and *morbidly obese* and instead favors terms such as *the person with obesity* and *the individual affected by obesity*. These are phrases that show respect and put the person before the disease. Table 6.1 provides the preferred terms and those that should be avoided.

While PFL has been adopted and promoted by major obesity organizations and has been emphasized in obesity education programs, many healthcare professionals find it difficult to consistently use it, even when they have been educated on its importance in reducing stigma and improving the patient encounter [8]. It is not uncommon to hear clinicians use the term *obese* in the medical literature, professional presentations, and clinical conversations. Even when professional organizations set the clear standard that all obesity education must use PFL and speakers agree to use it, there are still instances in which these speakers are not fully compliant. It is clear that more work needs to be done to not only increase awareness about PFL for obesity, but to increase its consistent use.

Table 6.1 Appropriate language

Preferred terms	Terms to avoid
Person/individual with obesity	Fat
Person/individual living with obesity	Obese
Increased BMI	Morbidly obese
Eating plan/eating habits	Heavy
Physical activity	Large size
	Diet
	Exercise

If you hear other clinicians or staff use terms such as *obese, morbidly obese*, or other derogatory terms, it is important to provide a respectful reminder of the need to use PFL at all times. This in-the-moment education will help shift the thinking and behavior of the members of the healthcare team. It is not uncommon to hear patients refer to themselves or others as *obese* or *morbidly obese*. If this happens during a clinician-patient discussion, take the opportunity to educate your patient about PFL and encourage its adoption. This new perspective will help your patients see themselves in a new light, one in which they put themselves before their disease and can begin to release their internalized bias and shame.

6.5.5   Patient Preference

Asking patients about their language preferences conveys respect and provides clinicians with the specific terms each patient is comfortable with. Direct questions such as, "As we talk about your weight, which types of words and language would be most comfortable for you?" are effective. Some patients will state their preferences, whereas others may not have considered the impact of language and need guidance and time to determine their preferences. The word obesity has different connotations to different people. Given the stigma surrounding obesity, the word itself may be uncomfortable for patients to speak and hear. If a patient is unsure about preferences, questions that provide education and contain options may help the patient sort it out. One example is: "Obesity is a clinical word, but some patients are uncomfortable with it and prefer terms such as excess weight, unhealthy weight, extra weight. Do you have a preference?" This approach normalizes the patients' discomfort, invites them to give it further thought, and establishes a collaborative partnership between clinician and patient.

In clinical literature and discussions, the phrases "obesity is a disease" and "the disease of obesity" are often used with the goal of framing obesity as a health condition rather than a lifestyle choice. While these phrases are much needed in professional discussions, they may be uncomfortable for patients if used during clinician-patient discussions. Some patients feel relief when they hear "obesity is a disease" or are told they have a disease, as they have longed to have it identified as a health issue rather than a personal failing or lifestyle choice, whereas others are uncomfortable with the reference that they have a "disease." A sensitive approach is to refer to obesity as a *chronic health condition* and avoid using the word *disease* in clinician-patient discussions. If desired, you can wait until the discussion has progressed and then ask about preference, by asking the following: "When I discuss obesity with other clinicians, I refer to it as a disease to educate and reinforce that it is a health issue, not a personal choice. Some patients are uncomfortable with hearing the word disease in reference to their weight, while others feel relief. Some feel both. What is your preference?" This question not only invites your patients to explore their thoughts and feelings and better understand their own experience, it empowers them to speak their own truth. It communicates to patients that you are knowledgeable about obesity and that you are leading and advocating for them. Furthermore, it sends the message that you are on the patient's side, which is much needed given the weight bias that patients have experienced in healthcare.

All of these concepts—the value of building a partnership, seeking the patient's perspective, selecting appropriate patients, and the need to use respectful, non-biased language while keeping the conversation focused on health in a manner that will benefit the patient in the long-term—provide a framework from which conversation can begin. Two evidence-based theoretical frameworks, Motivational Interviewing (MI) and the 5As of obesity counseling, provide further guidance on how to conduct conversations that incorporate these concepts.

6.6   Motivational Interviewing

Motivational Interviewing (MI) is an evidence-based counseling approach that is used by clinicians when discussing health conditions for which behavior change is needed for successful management [9]. When compared to traditional advice giving, MI has been shown to be superior in the treatment of a broad range of physiologic and psychologic conditions and has been effective in improving health behaviors that have led to smoking cessation, cholesterol reduction, blood pressure reduction, improvements in eating and physical activity, and reductions in alcohol use [10]. Because obesity outcomes rely more on patient behaviors than clinician recommendations, an approach that effectively contributes to behavior change is needed. MI has been shown to be effective when counseling patients on weight and obesity, as it leads to changed behavior [11, 12].

This empathic person-centered style of therapeutic communication emerged as the psychologist William Miller became more attuned to the elements of his counseling that evoked change. In a particularly poignant moment, while demonstrating his structured behavioral approach for treating problem drinking to psychologists in Norway, he recognized that it wasn't the techniques he employed that were beneficial, but rather the empathy he conveyed and the way in which it strengthened motivation and reduced resistance [13]. After returning home he constructed a model and created clinical guidelines for MI, which were first published in 1983. Since that time, MI has been increasingly utilized by clinicians in the treatment of addiction and in the management of health conditions, particularly those that are chronic in nature, as it elicits behavior change that improves health outcomes and improves clinician-patient relationships [9].

MI is a clinical style that integrates person-centered empathy with behavioral therapy techniques, with a focus on developing and strengthening a collaborative clinician-patient relationship and eliciting patients' motivation to make behavior changes that promote health [9]. Given the predominance of advice-giving that clinicians have traditionally engaged in when discussing weight and obesity with patients and the negative impact it has had on those patients' health, a clinical conversation style that builds the therapeutic alliance and leads to improved health behaviors is much needed.

MI is derived from social-cognitive theory that applies the processes of attribution, cognitive dissonance, and self-efficacy [14]. It focuses on creating a clinician-patient relationship from which MI can be utilized to bring about behavior change that improves health. The relationship is founded on the concepts of collaboration, evocation, and autonomy [15], which are needed to build a trusting relationship that focuses on the patient's goals, rather than the clinician's goals. This relational approach conceptualizes motivation as something that is derived from the interpersonal process, rather than a personality trait of the patient [14]. The resultant change is attributed to the synergy of the relationship. Cognitive dissonance is created through contrasting the current behavior with its negative consequences. Through the application of empathic processes, utilization of the social psychological principles of motivation, and the provision of objective feedback, the dissonance is channeled towards behavior change that promotes self-efficacy [14]. The objective of MI is not to solve the problem, but to assist patients in believing that change is possible. MI shifts clinician thinking from one of advice giving to skillful reflective listening.

MI identifies, explores, and resolves patients' ambivalence about changing behavior. Ambivalence—feeling two seemingly opposite ways about making a change—is a natural part of the behavior change process. The clinician's role is to attune to the patient's ambivalence and explore it in a manner that makes it more explicit and understandable to both parties. This is accomplished by evoking patients' verbalized motivations for change, known as "change talk", as well as their resistance to making that change, which is called "sustain talk." Once it has been voiced by the patient, the clinician amplifies and reflects the change talk, which further strengthens it. It is powerful and change-promoting when patients hear themselves argue for change, which is a guiding principle of MI. When the "sustain talk" argument has been identified and verbalized, the clinician conveys empathy for that position, rather than pushing or arguing against it, as confrontation has been shown to be counterproductive [15]. When resistance has been voiced, the spirit of MI guides clinicians towards the expression of compassion and understanding, and the avoidance of confrontation. When clinician responses are consistent with the spirit of MI, patient change talk significantly increases and sustain talk decreases. As the patient voices desire, ability, reasons, and need for change, and sufficient motivation is apparent, the clinician intervenes in a manner that strengthens the patient's commitment and converts motivation into specific goals and plans [13]. This is the fertile soil from which change takes place.

6.7 The "Spirit" of Motivational Interviewing

MI is intended to help clinicians create a style of conversation, rather than provide them with techniques. Clinicians are most effective when they incorporate the spirit of MI into their approach and focus on their "way of being", as opposed to following a step-by-step formula of techniques. One of the tenets of MI is to build rapport in the initial stages of the clinician-patient relationship and to maintain the rapport as the relationship progresses [16]. The "spirit" of MI is comprised of three key elements: collaboration, evocation, and autonomy [9].

6.7.1 Collaboration

A collaborative clinician-patient relationship is foundational to the success of MI. Such a relationship relies on the creation of a partnership that is grounded in the perspectives and experiences of the patient, rather than positioning the clinician as the expert [9]. Because it is not a hierarchical relationship, decisions are made collaboratively. And because the clinician is not positioned as the expert, it prevents the patient from being a passive participant while the clinician directs the patient's behavior. It also reduces confrontation, which is likely to elicit defensiveness and resistance from the patient [9].

6.7.2 Evocation

The spirit of MI seeks to evoke the patient's motivation and resources for change and connect them to the patient's personal goals, values, aspirations, and dreams [9]. It requires clinicians to refrain from imposing their opinions or attempting to convince patients to change and to instead draw out the patient's motivators and skills for change. Unless the motivation comes from the patient, it will not result in lasting change.

6.7.3 Autonomy

The power for true change resides in the patient. When practicing the spirit of MI, clinicians accept the decisions patients make and detach themselves from the outcomes, while maintaining a caring presence [9]. Paradoxically, this stance is one that is more likely to facilitate behavior change. When clinicians communicate respect for their patients' autonomy, they increase the chance that patients will exercise that autonomy for their own benefit. Honoring patients' autonomy strengthens their ability to harness their power to make choices that promote health.

Incorporating these three elements into clinical conversation is in stark contrast to the traditional view that the clinician is the expert, and the patient is the passive recipient. Yet given the evidence that communicating from a position of expert by advising patients to lose weight contributes to patients disengaging from not only the clinician-patient relationship, but from seeking healthcare altogether, a new approach is needed [1]. The elements of collaboration, evocation, and autonomy provide a more effective approach.

6.8   The Principles of Motivational Interviewing

In *Motivational Interviewing in Health Care: Helping Patients Change Behavior*, Rollnick et al. [9] provide the four guiding principles of MI, which are: (1) resist the righting reflex, (2) understand your patient's motivation, (3) listen to your patient, (4) empower your patient. These four principles—resist, understand, listen, empower—can be expressed in the acronym RULE [9].

6.8.1   *Resist the Righting Reflex*

Individuals typically enter healthcare professions to heal and lead people towards better health. These inclinations contribute to a "righting reflex" in which they automatically or reflexively step in to correct their patients' course when they see that they are headed down an unhealthy path [9]. When this occurs, it can have a paradoxical effect on their patients' motivation by evoking resistance and strengthening their argument against change. Therefore, it is incumbent upon clinicians to recognize and resist this tendency to step in and course correct. When the conversation becomes one in which the clinician is attempting to persuade the patient to change and is arguing with the patient about the best course, the righting reflex is at play. When the clinician is employing the spirit of MI, it is the patient who will voice the case for change, not the clinician [9].

6.8.2   *Understand Your Patient's Motivation*

Without an understanding of what is important to their patients, clinicians will not be able to strengthen their patients' change talk [9]. Because motivation is discovered and strengthened through interpersonal processes, inquiry about patients' concerns, values, and motivations not only provides clinicians with valuable information, it is a therapeutic intervention in its own right. Although such an inquiry may sound like a time-consuming endeavor, it may actually be one that saves time. Asking patients what they want to change and how they might make that change can be accomplished in a far shorter amount of time than trying to convince patients to change and then attempting to force a strategy. When motivation comes from the patient, it is more likely that the patient will make the changes necessary to improve health.

6.8.3   Listen to Your Patient

Listening is a necessary component of any type of effective conversation. The collaborative approach of MI recognizes that patients are the experts on themselves and that most of their answers reside within them [9]. The clinician's role is to ask evocative questions and listen with empathic interest for those answers. It's a sign of engagement when the patient is talking more than the clinician. When clinicians listen well and their patients feels heard, the relationship is strengthened. Quality listening is about more than hearing the words that are spoken, it is about hearing the messages and feelings that lie beneath those words. When clinicians listen for deeper meaning and themes, they are in a position to reflect on their impressions and share them with their patients, increasing both parties' understanding of the patients' truth—their motivations, their insights about what is needed, and their commitment to making the necessary changes. This type of listening relieves the clinician from having to provide all the answers, prevents resistance, and ultimately saves time. A good rule of thumb is for clinicians to listen more than they talk.

6.8.4   Empower Your Patient

The principle of empowerment is vital to helping patients take an active interest in their health, as the best outcomes are seen when patients are actively engaged in their own care [9]. The clinicians' role is to facilitate their patients' ability to locate and amplify their motivation, and then guide them in translating it into meaningful, consistent action. While clinicians are often clear on *why* change is needed, it is the patients who knows best about *how* it can be accomplished. Clinicians empower their patients when they invite them to tap into their own strengths and resources and support them in applying those strengths and resources towards the betterment of their own health. Providing hope that change is possible and conveying faith that patients have the capacity to make the needed changes are empowering actions. When clinicians acknowledge and celebrate their patients' autonomy, their patients feel empowered.

6.9   Bringing MI Principles to Life

The four guiding principles—resist the righting reflex, understand your patient's motivation, listen to your patient, empower your patient—paint a picture of two people interacting in a manner that looks and feels like dancing, not wrestling [9]. In order to create interactions that evoke images of two partners gliding across the dance floor, clinicians need a set of strategic actions, as well as specific skills, known as micro-counseling techniques.

6.10 Strategic Actions

There are four strategic actions that you can take to assist your patients in locating their motivation and putting it into action. Those actions are: (1) express empathy, (2) support self-efficacy, (3) roll with resistance, (4) develop discrepancy. These actions are ones that ensure your interactions with your patients will be aligned with the spirit and principles of MI.

6.10.1 Express Empathy

Empathy is the ability to enter into and understand the thoughts, experiences, and feelings of another person—to see the world through their eyes. Empathy is not the same as agreement, it is the ability to step into the experience of another person in order to understand it better. When you express empathy for your patients' thoughts and feelings, they will feel heard and understood and are likely to share themselves in deeper, more honest ways. Comments such as, "I understand how frustrated you feel," and "Your perspective makes sense," are expressions of empathy.

6.10.2 Support Self-Efficacy

Self-efficacy is a belief that one has the strength and capacity to successfully change. Without it, change is impossible. Most patients have likely made numerous attempts to change a problematic behavior or implement a new health behavior and not been successful, leaving them discouraged and questioning their ability to make the necessary changes. That is why it is vital that clinicians communicate their belief that their patients are capable of making the changes they desire. One strategy is to identify and highlight the skills and strengths that your patients already possess. Linking their ability to change and be effective in other areas of their health and life, provides them with the hope that they can access those strengths to make the change that lies in front of them. Examples of comments that support self-efficacy are: "You consistently take your blood pressure medications, I know you will be able to add this new medication to your routine," and "When you face a challenge at work, you stay with it until it is resolved. I know you will be able to apply that strength to this new health challenge."

6.10.3 Roll with Resistance

Resistance arises from a patient's ambivalence about change or when there is a conflict between the perspective of the patient and that of the clinician. It may also arise any time the patient feels an impingement on, or loss of, autonomy. If this occurs, it is strategic to roll with it rather than confront it. Because the goal is to dance, not wrestle, clinicians must de-escalate the situation in order to preserve the relationship and release patients from feeling the need to defend their position. If you do not roll with it, your patients are likely to strengthen their arguments not to change. When you invite your patients to define the problem and what can be done to solve it, rather than impose your perspectives, the likelihood of resistance arising is significantly reduced. In the event that you encounter a patient's resistance, you can de-escalate it with statements such as, "I sense that you feel that I have not fully heard your perspective. Please share your position again."

6.10.4   Develop Discrepancy

By identifying and leveraging the discrepancy between patients' goals and current actions, you can strengthen patients' motivation to change. Helping patients to see how their current behaviors are in conflict with their goals, values, and dreams has the power to increase their motivation and move them closer to making changes that are aligned with those goals, values, and dreams. Developing discrepancy is more of a process than a one-time action, as it takes time for patients to fully recognize that their behaviors may be moving them away from their goals, rather than towards them. While this is an important strategic action, clinicians need to ensure that it does not interfere with the principles of MI. When skillfully done, it will not induce resistance. An example of a reflection that illuminates discrepancy while maintaining the therapeutic relationship is: "You have expressed your desire to increase your stamina, yet you are struggling to walk regularly. What do you think is needed to make the change you desire?"

6.11   Micro Counseling Techniques

When utilizing MI, clinicians can employ micro-counseling techniques that will elicit the necessary information and motivation that is needed in an effective patient encounter. These techniques—open-ended questions, affirmations, reflections, and summaries—create the acronym OARS. Not only does OARS provide clinicians with specific behaviors, it summarizes the concepts of MI.

6.11.1   Open-Ended Questions

Open-ended questions require more than a yes or no response. They invite deeper thinking that leads to forward momentum. When patients elaborate on both their reasons for and the possibility of change, they become more attuned to what is motivating them to take action. Exploring one's own thought processes and behaviors can provide clarity about what is important and what is needed next. Open-ended questions facilitate patient engagement in the treatment. An example of an open-ended questions is: "What would it take to regularly get more sleep?"

6.11.2   *Affirmations*

Affirmations are statements that recognize and reinforce patients' strengths and how they can be utilized to facilitate positive change. They provide patients with the opportunity to see themselves in a more favorable manner and recognize that change is possible. This is particularly important if prior attempts have been unsuccessful. In order to be effective, affirmations need to be both relevant and genuine. Affirmations support self-efficacy. "You handled that challenge with courage. You stayed with it even when it was difficult."

6.11.3   *Reflections*

Reflective listening expresses empathy, making it crucial to effective MI. Effective reflections capture the essence of what the clinician has observed in the patient's body language, tone, and choice of words, and integrates them with the clinician's intuition and perceptions. This is a more challenging skill to master as it requires you to be attuned to the underlying thoughts and feelings that the patient may not be aware of. Reflections help patients clarify their reasons for and against change and illuminate the discrepancies in their thinking. Reflection may be as simple as repeating patients' words back to them or re-stating them in a manner that captures the deeper message you heard. An example of the latter scenario is: "You care deeply about preventing future health problems."

6.11.4   *Summaries*

Summarizing statements typically take place at the end of an appointment but may be utilized for transitions during the appointment. If a patient veers off topic, summarizing statements can be used to redirect the patient back to the topic at hand. Summaries call attention to the important elements of the discussion but may also highlight both sides of the patient's ambivalence or develop discrepancy. When the topics discussed have elicited strong emotions, summarizing statements provide the patient with a framework from which to think about what has been discussed and felt, and provide emotional closure before the patient reenters the outside world. A summary serves to shift attention from past challenges to the opportunities that lie ahead. It establishes metrics and outlines the next step. Summaries ensure that the clinician and the patient are both on the same page. An example of a summarizing statement that redirects the patient back to the topic being discussed is: "You came in today with the goal of discussing your eating plan, but we have spent the last five minutes discussing your co-worker. Let's shift back to your eating plan." An example of a summarizing statement at the end of an appointment is: "Today you made a commitment to menu plan and grocery shop every Saturday in order to stay on your eating plan."

6.12   The 5As

The 5As model provides an effective framework for counseling patients and has been used universally to teach clinicians how to encourage behavior change in their patients [17]. It was first developed by the U.S. Department of Health and Human Services as a framework for smoking cessation [17] and was informed by the trans-theoretical model of behavior change by Prochaska and DiClemente [18]. The model is used in Australia for smoking, alcohol, and physical activity counseling [19] and in Canada and other countries for obesity counseling [20]. The original 5As model was modified by the Canadian Obesity Network, now known as Obesity Canada, for the purpose of obesity counseling and is rooted in behavior change theory—self management, support, readiness, assessment, behavior modification, and self-efficacy enhancement [20]. It has been shown to be an effective framework from which to counsel patients about their weight [11, 21].

The 5As model has five elements—ask, assess, advise, agree, assist—that work well with the MI approach to conversation. While MI provides guidance on the style of conversation, the 5As model provides structure by identifying the phases and tasks that are required to move the conversation from inquiry to action. MI principles and techniques are incorporated into the conversation that takes place within the structure of the 5As. As with MI, the 5As model is patient-centered and emphasizes the importance of a collaborative clinician-patient relationship. It also supports the guiding concepts of focusing on health, focusing on the long-game, and using appropriate language.

The 5As model provides a time-efficient structure that can be used in busy practice settings, including primary care, specialty care, and other practice settings. This section will utilize the 5As structure to initiate sensitive conversations, move the patients who are ready into making a commitment to begin treatment, and provide the necessary support. For those who are not ready, guidance will be given on how to increase the likelihood that they will return for treatment in the future. While the 5As model identifies five distinctive phases, in real-life conversations these phases flow and blend. The delineation of each phase provides you with a more in-depth understanding of each phase and emphasizes its role in the overall approach.

The model can be adapted to fit into short appointments or expanded if more time is available. Unless the appointment was scheduled for the purpose of discussing obesity treatment, it is likely that the initial conversation will take place during an appointment that was scheduled for other reasons, making it more important that it be done efficiently and effectively. There may only be enough time to complete the first two As, ask and assess. When this is the case, obesity-specific follow-up will need to be scheduled to complete the conversation, whether it is with you or with a clinician to whom you are referring the patient. Although studies show that the 5As are effective in primary care only when clinicians include every phase in a single conversation [22], this is difficult to achieve in most practice settings due to time limitations and patient readiness factors, making it necessary to move beyond the perspective that everything needs to be discussed in one appointment [17].

6.12.1 Ask

In this stage of the conversation, the focus is on asking questions and minimizing statements. Some questions will be open-ended while others may only generate one-word answers. Both types are important, as they provide clinicians with information that will determine how to direct the conversation.

6.12.1.1 Ask Permission

When initiating discussions about weight, the first question should be one that asks patients for their permission to discuss weight. This approach differs from the initiation of discussions about other health issues, which do not typically involve asking for permission. Because weight is a sensitive topic and because many patients have received unsolicited advice to lose weight from clinicians in the past, asking permission sets the tone for a patient-centered discussion that honors patients' autonomy. The act of asking permission demonstrates a level of respect that many with obesity have not experienced in healthcare settings.

Examples of initial questions are:

- Do I have your permission to discuss your weight?
- Would it be alright if we discuss your weight?
- May I talk to you about your weight?
- Would you be open to a conversation about your weight?

If the patient agrees, the conversation should proceed. If not, it is best to respect the patient's wishes. It is advisable to acknowledge that respect with a statement such as, "I respect your wishes. If you are open to a discussion in the future, please let me know. I want you to know that the door is always open."

6.12.1.2   Ask About Readiness

Once permission has been obtained, the next questions should explore readiness.
Examples of questions that explore readiness are:

- Do you have any concerns about your weight?
- Do you have any concerns about how your weight affects your health?
- Do you have any concerns about your weight and your quality of life?
- Do you feel ready to work on your weight?
- How important is it to you to work on your weight?
- Would you be willing to discuss strategies to manage your weight?
- Are you open to discussing strategies to manage your weight?
- Would it be okay if I helped you manage your weight?
- Are you interested in discussing weight management strategies with me?

Although statements should be minimized, it can be beneficial for clinicians to share that they have knowledge about weight management and obesity, and/or treatment resources prior to asking questions about readiness. Such statements communicate that the clinician understands the complexities of weight issues and is someone patients can trust to provide accurate information and treatment resources, as opposed to the simplistic solutions that many have received in the past. Based on prior experiences, patients may be unwilling to continue the discussion, even if they are ready and willing to address their weight. Again, it is advisable to respect their wishes.

Examples of statements that are followed by questions that explore readiness are:

- I understand the complexities of weight. Would you be willing to discuss strategies with me?
- I can help you with your weight. Are you interested in discussing strategies with me?
- I've completed additional education on weight issues. Would you be willing to discuss strategies with me?
- I am sensitive to the challenges of weight management. Would you be willing to discuss strategies with me?

Readiness to Change

Patient responses provide information about their readiness to change. Readiness will run the spectrum from no interest to fully ready to commit to change. Prochaska's Stages of Change model identifies the five stages of change—precontemplation, contemplation, preparation, action, maintenance—which can assist you in identifying your patients' readiness to change [18]. Figure 6.1 provides further detail about the stages.

Patients in the precontemplation stage are not ready and may not be interested in further discussion. However, some may be interested and will accept your offer. The

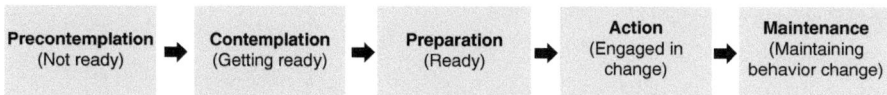

Fig. 6.1 Transtheoretical model of change (Adapted from: Prochaska JO, DiClemente CC. Stages and processes of self-change of smoking: toward an integrative model of change. J Consult Clin Psychol. 1983;51(3):390–5)

tone of the conversation and the information they receive may move them from precontemplation to contemplation. Those in the contemplation stage have an awareness that their weight is an issue and are considering taking action. Some may be ready to move into action, while others may not be there yet. If the patient isn't interested in pursuing it at this time, that should be respected.

However, it is important to invite patients to revisit the topic at a later date and provide information that will help move them to the next stage, such as brochures, links to websites that provide accurate information about obesity and evidence-based treatment options, as well as your contact information in the case that they desire further resources and support.

- I hear that you are not interested at this time. We can discuss this again when you feel ready. I have treatment options and resources when that time comes. Do you have any questions before we end this topic?
- I don't have the sense that this is something you are ready to embark on at this time. Is that correct?
- Weight management is challenging and it's important to be ready. We can revisit this at a later date. Perhaps you will feel differently as time passes or your circumstances change. Feel free to contact me when you are ready. Do you have any questions before we end this topic?
- I can see that you have other priorities at this time. You are welcome to contact me when your circumstances change. Do you have any questions before we end this topic?

Asking patients if they have any further questions provides them with the opportunity to clarify anything that is confusing and seek further information. It also provides them with a chance to evaluate your trustworthiness and commitment to a respectful clinician-patient relationship, which, based on prior experiences, they may be skeptical of.

When a patient chooses not to further the conversation or pursue treatment at the time the topic is broached, it is not a failure. An important health issue has been raised, which will not only help the patient make a deeper connection between weight and health, it will set the stage for further conversation. Having their wishes respected strengthens the therapeutic relationship.

Patients in the preparation stage are ready for change. Once you have obtained their permission to discuss weight, you can move into the next stage—assess.

6.12.2 Assess

The information gleaned from asking about interest and readiness leads naturally to the next stage—assess—which involves assessing health status. The assessment includes BMI, obesity stage, and identification of weight related risk factors and complications. BMI and obesity-related risk factors and complications may already be available in the medical record and may have been what prompted the clinician to initiate the conversation in the first place. If this information is not available, it can be assessed at this point if time permits.

The diagnosis and assessment should be recorded in the patient record. Even when obesity has been diagnosed, it is not always recorded in the record. One study looked at nearly 6200 health records in a primary care teaching practice and only 21.1% of patients with overweight or obesity had the diagnosis recorded in the chart [23].

6.12.3 Advise

In this phase of the discussion, clinicians provide education about the chronic, relapsing nature of obesity, the health benefits of a modest weight loss of 5–10%, the need for a long-term treatment strategy, and available treatment options. This education should include a personalized assessment of the patient's health status and how treatment can reduce risk and improve health. Before offering treatment recommendations, it is best to determine if the patient is interested in pursuing treatment by asking questions such as:

- Now that you have more information about what is involved, are you interested in discussing treatment options?
- Based on your understanding, would you like to discuss treatment options?
- Are you interested in pursuing treatment?
- Would you like me to recommend treatment options?

The answers to these questions will indicate whether or not the patient is ready to take action or would prefer to contemplate treatment or defer it to a later date. If the patient chooses not to pursue treatment, treatment information and resources should be provided, as well as an invitation to return when the patient is ready or if any questions arise in the interim. If the patient is agreeable, follow-up should be scheduled in 3–6 months so that the discussion can be revisited. Knowing that there will be further discussion increases the likelihood that the topic will remain active in the patient's mind.

When patients choose to pursue treatment, the conversation moves into the next phase: agree.

6.12.4 *Agree*

In this phase the clinician and patient agree that treatment is advisable, and realistic treatment goals are agreed upon. Treatment goals should be formulated collaboratively, rather than being imposed on the patient by the clinician. Patients are the ones who will be doing the hard work of behavior change and treatment plan implementation, so it is necessary for treatment goals to reflect their priorities and preferences. Many patients have unrealistic expectations about weight loss, so it is important to agree on an initial 5–10% loss and emphasize the physical and mental health benefits of a modest loss. Because weight regulation is complex and influenced by many factors, some of which are out of the patient's control, the conversation should focus on behavioral changes, rather than specific weight goals. Research shows that patients become discouraged if they don't meet their goals, reinforcing the importance of focusing primarily on behavior changes [20].

If this is the initial weight discussion between you and the patient and there is little time remaining in the appointment, further discussion will need to be deferred to a follow-up appointment. If a follow-up appointment is not possible, the patient should be given referral sources with an agreement about the need to pursue treatment and the benefits of doing so.

6.12.5 *Assist*

Once there is agreement about the treatment goals and the benefits of pursuing treatment, the clinician assists the patient in identifying facilitators such as motivating factors, support systems and other resources as well as any social, medical, emotional, and economic barriers. Discussion about available treatment options and resources should occur, with the clinician assisting the patient in arranging follow-up. If you will be managing the obesity treatment, a plan will be made for obesity-specific appointments during which a more thorough evaluation will be conducted, and a treatment plan will be formulated and implemented. If the patient will be referred, then a clear plan for the next step should be given. Chapter 8 provides guidance on treatment options and resources.

6.13 Summary

Conversations about weight and obesity are most effective when the focus is on the patient's health. This is accomplished by building a respectful, collaborative clinician-patient partnership in which the patient's perspective is elicited and valued. Using appropriate, non-stigmatizing language, particularly PFL, is vital to ensuring that the conversation feels respectful to the patient. MI provides a framework for building this relationship and evokes the patient's own motivation. The 5As model provides the structure from which to move the conversation from initiation of the topic to the initiation of treatment and beyond. Discussions about obesity are not a one-time event; each conversation should set the stage for the next one.

References

1. Mensinger JL, Tylka TL, Calamari ME. Mechanisms underlying weight status and healthcare avoidance in women: a study of weight stigma, body-related shame and guilt, and healthcare stress. Body Image. 2018;25:139–47.
2. Bocquier A, Verger P, Basdevant A, Andreotti G, Baretge J, Villani P, et al. Overweight and obesity: knowledge, attitudes, and practices of general practitioners in France. Obes Res. 2005;13(4):787–95.
3. Campbell K, Engel H, Timperio A, Cooper C, Crawford D. Obesity management: Australian general practitioners' attitudes and practices. Obes Res. 2000;8(6):459–66.
4. Fogelman Y, Vinker S, Lachter J, Biderman A, Itzhak B, Kitai E. Managing obesity: a survey of attitudes and practices among Israeli primary care physicians. Int J Obes Relat Metab Disord. 2002;26(10):1393–7.
5. Brown I. Nurses' attitudes towards adult patients who are obese: literature review. J Adv Nurs. 2006;53(2):221–32.
6. Befort CA, Greiner KA, Hall S, Pulvers KM, Nollen NL, Charbonneau A, et al. Weight-related perceptions among patients and physicians: how well do physicians judge patients' motivation to lose weight? J Gen Intern Med. 2006;21(10):1086–90.
7. Amy NK, Aalborg A, Lyons P, Keranen L. Barriers to routine gynecological cancer screening for White and African-American obese women. Int J Obes. 2006;30(1):147–55.
8. Hauff C, Fruh SM, Sims BM, Williams SG, Herf C, Golden A, et al. Nurse practitioner students' observations of preceptor engagement in obesity management and weight bias: a mixed-methods approach. J Am Assoc Nurse Pract. 2020;32(7):520–9.
9. Rollnick S, Miller WR, Butler CC. Motivational interviewing in health care: helping patients change behavior. New York: The Guilford Press; 2008.
10. Rubak S, Sandbaek A, Lauritzen T, Christensen B. Motivational interviewing: a systematic review and meta-analysis. Br J Gen Pract. 2005;55(513):305–12.
11. Gudzune KA, Clark JM, Appel LJ, Bennett WL. Primary care providers' communication with patients during weight counseling: a focus group study. Patient Educ Couns. 2012;89(1):152–7.
12. Armstrong MJ, Mottershead TA, Ronksley PE, Sigal RJ, Campbell TS, Hemmelgarn BR. Motivational interviewing to improve weight loss in overweight and/or obese patients: a systematic review and meta-analysis of randomized controlled trials. Obes Rev. 2011;12(9):709–23.
13. Miller WR, Rose GS. Toward a theory of motivational interviewing. Am Psychol. 2009;64(6):527–37.
14. Miller WR. Motivational interviewing with problem drinkers. Behav Psychother. 1983;11(2):147–72.
15. Miller WR, Rollnick S. Motivational interviewing: helping people change. 3rd ed. New York: Guilford Press; 2013.
16. Tahan HA, Sminkey PV. Motivational interviewing: building rapport with clients to encourage desirable behavioral and lifestyle changes. Prof Case Manag. 2012;17(4):164–72; quiz 73–4.

17. Sturgiss E, van Weel C. The 5As framework for obesity management: do we need a more intricate model? Can Fam Physician. 2017;63(7):506–8.
18. Prochaska JO, DiClemente CC. Stages and processes of self-change of smoking: toward an integrative model of change. J Consult Clin Psychol. 1983;51(3):390–5.
19. Sim MG, Wain T, Khong E. Influencing behaviour change in general practice—part 1—brief intervention and motivational interviewing. Aust Fam Physician. 2009;38(11):885–8.
20. Vallis M, Piccinini-Vallis H, Sharma AM, Freedhoff Y. Clinical review: modified 5As: minimal intervention for obesity counseling in primary care. Can Fam Physician. 2013;59(1):27–31.
21. Washington Cole KO, Gudzune KA, Bleich SN, Bennett WL, Cheskin LJ, Henderson JL, et al. Influence of the 5A's counseling strategy on weight gain during pregnancy: an observational study. J Womens Health (Larchmt). 2017;26(10):1123–30.
22. Sherson EA, Yakes Jimenez E, Katalanos N. A review of the use of the 5A's model for weight loss counselling: differences between physician practice and patient demand. Fam Pract. 2014;31(4):389–98.
23. Cyr PR, Haskins AE, Holt C, Hanifi J. Weighty problems: predictors of family physicians documenting overweight and obesity. Fam Med. 2016;48(3):217–21.

Chapter 7
Clinical Scenarios

7.1 Introduction

This chapter will provide you with four clinical scenarios and five conversations that illustrate the concepts that have been covered in this book. Each conversation is followed by a discussion about the concepts and techniques that were incorporated into the conversation and how the style and substance of the conversation moved the patient closer towards improved health. Each clinician demonstrates how to build a strong and trusting clinician-patient partnership and how to set the stage for further conversations.

7.2 Clinical Scenario 1

Sadhavi is a 41 year-old Indian female with obesity (BMI 34.4) who is seeing her endocrine nurse practitioner for a follow-up after being diagnosed with type 2 diabetes a year ago. Diabetes is now under control, but she has elevated triglycerides, suppressed HDL-C, and elevated liver enzymes. Blood pressure is not fully controlled. She has a family history of type 2 diabetes, hypertension, and cardiovascular disease.

After reviewing labs and agreeing to continue the same treatment regimen, there are 5 min remaining in the appointment. The clinician decides to open a conversation about weight.

© Springer Nature Switzerland AG 2021

S. Christensen, *A Clinician's Guide to Discussing Obesity with Patients*,
https://doi.org/10.1007/978-3-030-69311-4_7

- Nurse Practitioner: "Now that your diabetes has improved, would it be alright if we discuss your weight?"
- Sadhavi: "Yes."
- Nurse Practitioner: "What are your thoughts about how your weight affects your health?"
- Sadhavi: "It slows me down. It's hard to keep up with my kids and I'm pretty sure it contributes to my knee pain. My grandmother needed kidney dialysis and I don't want that to happen to me."
- Nurse Practitioner: "It sounds like you are motivated to feel better and prevent future health problems."
- Sadhavi: "I am. I'm relieved that my diabetes numbers are good, but I think I would feel so much better if I lost some weight. I'm too young to feel this way."
- Nurse Practitioner: "I can help you with your weight. Would you be willing to come back for another appointment so we can talk more about it?"
- Sadhavi: "I've never had a medical professional offer that before. Do you really think you can help me?"
- Nurse Practitioner: "Weight issues are common, and we have more tools than ever to address them. I will tell you more at your next appointment."
- Sadhavi: "I've never thought about it that way before. I thought I had to figure it out on my own."
- Nurse Practitioner: "Here are some forms I'd like you to fill out. We'll review them together at your next appointment. They will help me understand more about how your weight has affected you and your health and what you have tried to manage it."
- Sadhavi: "I'll do it."
- Nurse Practitioner: "Do you have any questions before we end?"
- Sadhavi: "I don't. I'll see you next time."

7.2.1 Discussion

This scenario demonstrates a smooth, successful conversation that resulted in Sadhavi agreeing to start obesity treatment. Having witnessed Sadhavi get her diabetes under control, the nurse practitioner saw an opportunity to address obesity. Because there were still metabolic concerns—elevated triglycerides, suppressed HDL-C and elevated liver enzymes—the nurse practitioner knew it was important to intervene to further improve metabolic health and prevent the development of obesity complications.

The nurse practitioner opened the conversation at the end of an appointment in which there was adequate time to begin the process of assessing Sadhavi's readiness. After seeking permission to discuss weight, the nurse practitioner asked an open-ended question *("What are your thoughts about how your weight affects your health?")* that kept the focus on health and elicited Sadhavi's perspective. Sadhavi's answer revealed her ability to connect her weight to her current health (her weight slows her down and contributes to knee pain) and her future health (she wants to prevent diabetes complications, which she's witnessed in a family member). These connections indicated her readiness for further conversation.

The nurse practitioner responded with a reflection *("It sounds like you are motivated to feel better and prevent future health problems.")*. Sadhavi confirmed that the reflection was correct and shared more about the factors that are motivating her, which are that she wants to keep up with her kids and feel more energetic. She also made a deeper connection between her weight and daily function and recognized that weight loss would make her feel better. Based on these readiness indicators, the nurse practitioner broached the topic of obesity treatment by first offering to be helpful and then directly asking Sadhavi if she would be willing to return for further discussion. Sadhavi's response ("I've never had a medical professional offer that before. Do you really think you can help me?") communicated her hope that the nurse practitioner might be helpful, to which the nurse practitioner responded with reassurance that obesity is common and treatable. Sadhavi's response ("I've never thought about it that way before. I thought I had to figure it out on my own.") indicated that Sadhavi has believed that she is solely responsible for managing her weight and has likely felt alone and overwhelmed by it. This response opened the door for the nurse practitioner to frame obesity as a health issue that they will tackle together. The nurse practitioner provided reassurance that this will be a collaborative partnership by telling Sadhavi that they will review the forms together so that the nurse practitioner can learn more about Sadhavi's experiences.

Throughout the conversation, the nurse practitioner used the principles of MI to build a respectful collaborative partnership in which Sadhavi's perspective and motivating factors were elicited and valued. When the nurse practitioner asked open-ended questions, they were focused on eliciting information that was pertinent to the topic and served to keep the conversation within the time available. The question, *"What are your thoughts about how your weight affects your health?"* invited Sadhavi to share her perspective within the scope of connecting weight and health. As Sadhavi shared her thoughts, her motivation was strengthened. The nurse practitioner understood the scope of what could be covered in a short period of time and limited the use of the 5As to ask and assess, while arranging for an obesity-specific follow-up appointment during which further discussion will take place.

When they meet for their first obesity specific appointment, the nurse practitioner has already gleaned valuable information about Sadhavi's motivating factors, her desire for health, and what is important to her. This will guide the remainder of the assessment and the formulation of the treatment plan, which will be personalized to what is motivating Sadhavi—feeling more energetic, reducing knee pain, and preventing diabetes complications.

7.3   Clinical Scenario 2

Eduardo is a 61 year-old Latino male who is visiting an orthopedic surgeon for the first time for severe right knee pain. He has obesity (BMI 44.1), hypertension and hyperlipidemia. He has a family history of obesity and cardiovascular disease. His father had a fatal myocardial infarction at age 64. This discussion begins after the surgeon has completed an evaluation of Eduardo's knee.

- Surgeon: "It looks like you have osteoarthritis in your knee. The cartilage in your joint has deteriorated and is what we call "bone on bone.' Given the severity, I recommend a total knee replacement. We can also discuss other treatment options, but they will only give you short-term pain relief and will not solve the issue."
- Eduardo: "I'm not too keen on surgery. What else have you got for me?"
- Surgeon: "I can inject a medication into the joint that will decrease inflammation and will likely provide some pain relief. Everyone has a different response, from minimal to significant pain relief that lasts a few weeks to several months. There is no way to know what your response will be, but most people get some relief."
- Eduardo: "What happens after it wears off?"
- Surgeon: "We can give you another injection, but you can only receive a maximum of three injections per year. Most people get more relief from their first injection and varied responses with additional injections. You will ultimately require a knee replacement."
- Eduardo: "Okay, I'll take the injection."
- Surgeon: "Besides cortisone and surgery, there is another factor that would improve the situation with your knee. Would you be willing to discuss your weight?"
- Eduardo: "Okay."
- Surgeon: "Body weight puts pressure on weight bearing joints such as knees. A modest weight reduction would relieve some of that pressure. It would also reduce your risk of other health problems such as cardiovascular disease. I can refer you to an obesity specialist who will do a full evaluation and develop a personalized plan. Would you like me to give you her contact information?"
- Eduardo: "No thanks. I'm not interested. Let's do the shot."
- Surgeon: "I respect your decision. If things change for you, please contact me and I'll give you the name of the specialist. The front desk will schedule your injection. I'll see you then."
- Eduardo: "Thanks."

Two weeks later Eduardo returned for his first cortisone injection.

7.3.1   Discussion

This conversation was well-placed at the end of an appointment for which Eduardo was receiving treatment for an obesity complication, although it did not result in him pursuing treatment. Throughout the conversation the surgeon focused on health and considered the long game. Recognition that obesity was impacting Eduardo's osteoarthritis and that his cardiovascular risk is elevated due to obesity and his father's early death from a heart attack prompted the surgeon to raise the topic.

The surgeon initiated the topic respectfully by asking for permission to discuss weight, which is the standard of care and is a favorable way to establish a respectful relationship with a new patient. Due to time constraints, the surgeon did not ask Eduardo open-ended questions to learn more about his perspective on his weight and health. The surgeon focused on providing Eduardo with an explanation of the benefits of weight reduction that were tailored to his current complaint and cardio-vascular risk and offered a treatment option. When Eduardo declined, the surgeon honored Eduardo's autonomy, preserved the relationship, and kept the door open for future discussion. Eduardo didn't provide his rationale for declining the knee replacement or obesity treatment and because time was limited, the surgeon did not pursue it, which is a real-world clinical reality. The surgeon made the assessment that Eduardo is not ready for treatment and resisted the righting reflex by not trying to convince him otherwise. Despite the constraints, the surgeon played the long game by building the partnership and planting seeds for future conversations.

7.3.2   Four Months Later

- Surgeon: "Hi Eduardo, how is the pain in your knee since your injection?"
- Eduardo: "It felt better for a couple of months, but now it hurts more than ever."
- Surgeon: "Last time we discussed the possibility of a knee replacement. Is that something you'd be willing to discuss at this point?"
- Eduardo: "Yeah, maybe. I don't want to do it but I'm realizing I need to. I'm worried that it won't go well. My buddy had complications when he got his new knee. I don't want that to happen to me."
- Surgeon: "We know that surgery outcomes are better when patients are below a specific weight threshold. Would you be open to a discussion about your weight?"
- Eduardo: "I guess so. Last time you wanted to send me to a specialist, but I didn't want to go."
- Surgeon: "I recall that. What were your reasons?"

- Eduardo: "I had a looming deadline at work and I just didn't have the bandwidth for one more thing. Besides, I've lost weight so many times and I always gain it back. I don't want to feel like a failure again."
- Surgeon: "Many people struggle with losing weight and keeping it off. Science has evolved and we now have a better understanding of the complexity, as well as more effective treatments."
- Eduardo: "What kind of treatments?"
- Surgeon: "The obesity specialist I mentioned last time will do a thorough evaluation and give you a personalized plan that includes nutrition, physical activity guidelines, behavioral strategies, and possibly medication."
- Eduardo: "Okay, I'll give it a try. I can't live with this pain and I want my surgery to be successful. But it's not just my knee I'm concerned about, my dad died of a heart attack when he was three years older than I am now. He had a weight problem too."
- Surgeon: "It's good to hear that your health is important to you and that you want to prevent the complications that your dad experienced. Obesity has a genetic component, which has likely contributed to your challenges with it. The obesity specialist will want to know more about your health goals and what is motivating you to address your weight, so that the two of you can develop a personalized treatment strategy."
- Eduardo: "That's good to know."

7.3.3 Discussion

In this conversation, the surgeon built on topics from the previous discussion and Eduardo was more responsive. This is likely a result of the tone of the previous conversation, which appears to have moved Eduardo from precontemplation to contemplation. He disclosed his reasons for declining a knee replacement and obesity treatment and the surgeon skillfully linked both health concerns in a manner that led to Eduardo committing to obesity treatment and preparing for a knee replacement.

Early in the conversation Eduardo shared his concern about developing complications after knee replacement surgery. The surgeon wove the connection between obesity and surgical complications together with the statement and question, *"We know that surgery outcomes are better when patients are below a specific weight threshold. Would you be open to a discussion about your weight?"* Once Eduardo opened up about his decision not to pursue obesity treatment, the surgeon invited further disclosure with a non-judgmental affirmation of Eduardo's autonomy *("I recall that.")* followed by an open-ended question that invited him to share his perspective *("What were your reasons?")*. Eduardo shared his barriers, primarily that he was overwhelmed at the time of the last conversation and his prior difficulty with maintaining weight loss and fear of repeated failure. The surgeon's compassionate response (*"Many people struggle with losing weight and keeping it off. Science has evolved and we now have a better understanding of the complexity, as well as more effective treatments."*) normalized Eduardo's experience and provided him with hope about future endeavors. This elicited Eduardo's curiosity about the type of available treatments. After the surgeon emphasized the personalized approach to obesity treatment, Eduardo made a deeper connection between obesity and his cardiovascular risk and how weight reduction could improve his surgical outcome. These connections both revealed and strengthened his motivation to address his weight. This conversation moved Eduardo from considering obesity treatment (contemplation) to agreeing to it (preparation).

7.4   Clinical Scenario 3

Judith is a 67 year-old Caucasian female seeing her primary care physician assistant of 17 years for her annual wellness visit. She has obesity (BMI 42.6), prediabetes, atrial fibrillation (diagnosed 10 months ago), and a history of endometrial cancer at age 63. Judith was referred to a cardiologist for atrial fibrillation and was started on a beta blocker. In the past year she has gained 21 pounds, prediabetes has worsened, and triglycerides are now elevated. She has a family history of cardiovascular disease and Alzheimer's.

- Physician Assistant: "How have you been doing since you received your atrial fibrillation diagnosis?"
- Judith: "The whole thing has been shocking and scary. After getting through endometrial cancer, I thought I was done with health issues for a while. I don't want to have problems like this. I've got grandkids I want to see grow up!"
- Physician Assistant: "I hear how important your health is to you. How are you feeling now?"
- Judith: "I'm doing better now. When it first started, I was so exhausted. It's better now, but the new medication slows me down."
- Physician Assistant: "Beta-blockers are known for that. They also contribute to weight gain. Do I have your permission to discuss your weight?"
- Judith: "Yes. I know I've gained weight since all this happened. How much is it up?"
- Physician Assistant: "Twenty-one pounds in the last year."
- Judith: "Oh dear. How much do you think the medication is contributing?"
- Physician Assistant: "I don't know exactly. But we do know that carrying extra weight increases the risk and severity of atrial fibrillation."
- Judith: "Why didn't the cardiologist tell me that the medication would cause weight gain?"

- Physician Assistant: "I don't know, but I'm sorry that you weren't told. Unfortunately, some clinicians prescribe medications that cause weight gain and don't discuss it with their patients. I can understand why you are frustrated."
- Judith: "Well, I'm glad we're talking about it now."
- Physician Assistant: "I am too. Weight gain may also increase the risk of prediabetes progressing to diabetes."
- Judith: "I definitely don't want diabetes on top of everything else!
- Physician Assistant: Would you be interested in discussing strategies for weight loss?"
- Judith: "Yes, but I'm so overwhelmed with everything else that I don't know where to start."
- Physician Assistant: "I've completed specialized education in obesity treatment. Would you be willing to work with me to get your weight under control?"
- Judith: "Maybe. What does it involve?"
- Physician Assistant: "I work with a multi-disciplinary team here at the clinic. I will manage your treatment, but you will see others on the team who also have specialized education. We will create a personalized plan that includes nutrition, physical activity, behavioral strategies, and possibly medication. We will meet regularly to implement and reinforce the plan."
- Judith: "I didn't know so much was available. I hope it's not too hard. I'm really taxed with everything else going on in my life."
- Physician Assistant: "We'll take it step by step. Our first goal is to stop further weight gain. Once we've accomplished that task, we can talk about your next goal."
- Judith: "That sounds reasonable. How do we get started?"

7.4.1 Discussion

This conversation took place within the context of an established warm, collaborative partnership between Judith and her physician assistant. Because of their history, the physician assistant had relational capitol to spend in the service of Judith's health. Having made the connection between obesity and Judith's health concerns—atrial fibrillation, prediabetes, hypertriglyceridemia, a history of endometrial cancer, and a family history of cardiovascular disease and Alzheimer's—the physician assistant entered the conversation with the intention of spending that capitol by addressing Judith's obesity. Based on previous interactions, the physician assistant was fairly confident that Judith would be receptive. The conversation was successful in that the collaborative partnership deepened and Judith agreed to return for obesity treatment with enhanced motivation to improve her health.

The physician assistant began the conversation by discussing a recent and serious health concern—atrial fibrillation—that is impacted by obesity and for which the treatment (a beta blocker) has worsened obesity. This elicited Judith's concern about her health and what is motivating her to improve it—wanting to see her grandkids grow up. The physician assistant responded with a reflection *("I hear how important your health is to you.")* followed by a focused open-ended question *(How are you feeling now?")*. Knowing that beta blockers contribute to weight gain and fatigue, the physician assistant designed the question to both gather information about the impact of the medication on Judith's daily functioning and lead the conversation to her weight. The question was effective and led Judith to further reflect on the medication's effects. The physician assistant informed Judith about the weight gaining effects of beta blockers with the goal of helping her feel less responsible for the gain. Hopefully, this will reduce the likelihood that Judith will get caught in self-blame and will increase her ability to focus on improving her health. Judith was understandably upset that the cardiologist didn't discuss the potential for weight gain with beta blockers. Her anger is felt by others who have unknowingly taken medications that cause or worsen obesity and have been left alone to deal with the effects, and worse yet, feel solely responsible for their weight gain. The physician assistant added an additional incentive by explaining the connection between weight gain and the progression of prediabetes to diabetes, which Judith was quick to pick up on.

Based on Judith's readiness indicators she was told about the physician assistant's specialized training in obesity management and was asked directly if she would be willing to work on her weight. At Judith's request, the physician assistant advised her about the comprehensive, personalized treatment structure, discussed the initial treatment goals, and provided reassurance that everything will happen step-by-step so that she won't get overwhelmed. Judith agreed to start treatment.

Throughout the conversation, the physician assistant kept the focus on health and used a conversational style that was aligned with the spirit of MI—collaboration, evocation, and autonomy. The physician assistant practiced the MI principles of understanding the patient's motivation, listening to the patient, and empowering the patient. The micro counseling techniques of OARS—open-ended questions, affirmations, reflections, and summaries—were used. The conversation followed the structure of the 5As. Although most of the conversation was spent asking and assessing, the physician assistant also advised, arranged, and assisted in order to lead the patient to the next step.

7.5 Clinical Scenario 4

Layla is a 47 year-old black female who is here to see her new primary care physician for her annual wellness visit. Her last annual was 2 years and 3 months ago, which was the last time she was seen by a healthcare provider or had any preventative screening. She has obesity (BMI 38.3), prediabetes, non-alcoholic fatty liver disease (NAFLD), and hypertension. She takes an anti-hypertensive medication but ran out several months ago. Blood pressure is elevated at this visit.

- Physician: "I'm glad you came in today. We got that pap done, I ordered your mammogram, and we'll get you back on your blood pressure medication."
- Layla: "Yeah, it feels good to have it done. I really didn't want to come but I needed my blood pressure pills. My uncle just had a stroke and I don't want that to happen to me."
- Physician: "You are wise to make the connection between high blood pressure and increased risk of stroke."
- Layla: "I like you better than the last doctor I saw here. She was always telling me that I need to lose weight. I haven't come back because I just didn't want to hear it. All she ever said was, 'You need to eat less and move more and then you will lose weight.' She had no idea how many times I've tried that or how hard it is to lose weight."
- Physician: "I hear how frustrating that was for you. Would you be comfortable discussing your weight with me?"
- Layla: "As long as you don't hassle me or tell me to try harder. If trying harder was the solution, I wouldn't have a weight problem."
- Physician: "What would you think about making an appointment to come back and discuss this further? Treatment has evolved, and I have some strategies that are safe and effective. This is rarely something people can do alone. Most need the support and expertise of a clinician who understands weight issues."
- Layla: "What kind of strategies?"
- Physician: "I will do a full assessment so that I can learn more about what has worked for you and what hasn't. Then we'll develop a personalized plan."
- Layla: "What will it involve?"
- Physician: "I will give you personalized recommendations for nutrition, physical activity, and other lifestyle modifications. We may consider FDA approved anti-obesity medications. We will work on it together and everything will be done one step at a time."
- Layla: "What about my prediabetes and fatty liver. That's what I'm most concerned about."
- Physician: "The treatment I'll recommend will improve both conditions. Treating obesity first often improves other health issues and reduces the risk of developing other problems."
- Layla: "Will I see you or someone else?"
- Physician: "I'll manage your treatment but will refer you to a dietician and will provide other resources that will support you."
- Layla: "Is she going to be one of those uptight dieticians who tells me to eat lettuce and push myself away from the table?"
- Physician: "No but I understand why you are concerned about that. She understands weight issues and will partner with you to create a plan that works for you."
- Layla: "That's good. I won't last long with someone who doesn't get it. I'll give it a try."

7.5.1 Discussion

This conversation demonstrates the ways in which biased experiences in healthcare leave scars that prevent patients from returning for preventative and follow-up care. This physician showed us how focusing on the patient's experience and perspective can begin to heal those scars by creating a positive, respectful experience in the here and now. In many ways, Layla was the ideal patient in that she was extremely forthright about the experiences she had with the previous clinician, how they kept her away, and what she needed from the physician and anyone to whom she might be referred. Although the conversation began with Layla saying she didn't want to be there, it ended with her agreeing to obesity treatment.

The physician set the tone for a collaborative partnership by commending Layla for coming in and summarizing what had already been accomplished in the appointment. This evoked Layla to reveal what had motivated her to schedule the appointment, which was her uncle's recent stroke and her desire to prevent one in herself. The physician further reinforced Layla's connection between hypertension and stroke, setting the stage to introduce the role of obesity treatment in controlling blood pressure and reducing stroke risk. Sensing safety and acceptance, Layla volunteered her reason for not returning for healthcare sooner—she was afraid of encountering a clinician who didn't understand obesity and who pushed unsolicited weight loss advice on her. The physician responded with empathy *(I hear how frustrating that was for you.)* and asked permission to discuss weight. Layla agreed, but set clear parameters: *"As long as you don't hassle me or tell me to try harder."* Layla further explained that she has tried to lose weight numerous times and hasn't been successful. Because previous weight loss attempts can be an indicator of current readiness, the physician asked Layla if she would be interested in discussing obesity treatment. The physician shared information about the availability of safe and effective treatments, emphasized that many people need the support of clinicians who understand obesity, and offered to provide personalized, stepwise treatment. Layla raised her concern about prediabetes and NAFLD, which were further indicators that she is motivated to improve her health. The physician connected obesity with both conditions and emphasized that treating obesity would improve all of the health issues that are concerning Layla. Upon learning that treatment would involve seeing a dietician, Layla made it clear that seeing a dietician who doesn't understand obesity won't work for her. The physician empathized with Layla's concern and reassured her that everyone on the treatment team understands the challenges of obesity and will collaborate with her.

This physician incorporated the concepts of MI and the structure of the 5As into the conversation. The physician's primary focus was to build a trusting clinician-patient partnership with Layla. Despite Layla's initial protest, she was surprisingly responsive to the physician's efforts. This serves as a reminder that we may discover patients who are more ready for us to initiate the conversation than they may appear initially. It emphasizes the importance of being curious and compassionate and showing empathy for the lived experiences of patients with obesity, especially those with visible scars from past interactions in healthcare settings.

7.6 Summary

In each scenario, the clinician sent the strong and powerful message: *"It's you and me against the disease."* The clinicians showed their patients that they were on their side by prioritizing the relationship and offering their empathy, curiosity, compassion, and steady presence. They were more concerned with creating a positive experience than trying to convince the patient to see their point of view. The concepts of MI and the structure of the 5As provided the framework from which these productive conversations took place.

Chapter 8
Taking the Next Step

8.1 Introduction

Each chapter of this book provides you with all of the elements you need to start productive conversations with your patients—conversations that will lead them to better health. This chapter summarizes what you've learned by reviewing the highlights of each chapter, which refreshes your knowledge and solidifies your ability to put your knowledge into practice. This chapter also provides you with an overview of what comes after you have successfully engaged your patients in taking the step into treatment. You will receive information that will guide you in educating patients about the disease of obesity and the need for long-term follow-up. You will learn more about the settings in which obesity is treated and how to refer to obesity specialists and bariatric surgery centers. For those who are interested in furthering their knowledge, additional educational resources will be provided.

8.2 What You've Learned

In Chap. 1 you learned that obesity is a chronic, progressive, relapsing disease that needs to be approached as any other chronic condition. Your deepened knowledge about the pathophysiology provides you with an enhanced understanding—one that is lacking in many clinicians—as to the numerous complexities, contributing factors, and the significant health risks of obesity. You are now aware that the goals of treatment are to improve health, reduce body weight, improve body composition, and improve quality of life. You know that when obesity is treated first, other conditions improve or resolve, and further complications may be prevented. You are keenly aware that the earlier the intervention, the better the outcome. All of this knowledge will prevent you from falling into treatment inertia and will mobilize you to address it with your patients.

© Springer Nature Switzerland AG 2021
S. Christensen, *A Clinician's Guide to Discussing Obesity with Patients*,
https://doi.org/10.1007/978-3-030-69311-4_8

In Chap. 2 we dove into the prevalence and seriousness of weight bias and how it plays out in every aspect of your patients' lives. You know that weight bias and stigma are at the root of why obesity is not recognized and treated as a disease. You learned how common it is in healthcare settings and how it negatively impacts your patients' physical and psychological health. Your knowledge about all the ways in which patients are stigmatized in healthcare settings expands your awareness about the need to identify and reduce weight bias in your practice setting and the importance of approaching your patients in an unbiased manner.

Chapter 3 provided you with strategies for reducing weight bias in healthcare, including tools that you can use to identify, explore, and manage your own weight bias. You received resources that will expand your understanding of obesity etiology and treatment. And you have a better understanding as to how this knowledge reduces weight bias. You also received additional educational resources on weight bias. You learned about the ways in which you can educate other members of the healthcare team and why it's important for you to be an agent for change. If you are an educator, you were given resources that can be used to incorporate obesity education into the curriculum and how doing so is vital to reducing weight bias in healthcare providers. Lastly you learned how to recognize and reduce internalized bias in your patients with the goal of improving their health.

Chapter 4 explored the numerous barriers that block you and your patients from having effective discussions about weight. We imagined that each barrier is a brick, and that one by one they build a wall which prevents clinicians and patients from engaging in productive conversations. You learned that many of the bricks are formed by a lack of clinical education about obesity and a lack of knowledge about strategies for discussing it with knowledge and sensitivity. But it isn't just a lack of education that adds bricks; time limitations, poor reimbursement, weight bias, and clinicians' fear of making patients uncomfortable are also barriers. Patient barriers were also explored, many of which are rooted in internalized weight bias. You were shown how to identify your patients' internalized bias and recognize its role in preventing productive discussion. After an exploration of each barrier, you learned how to dismantle the wall, brick by brick, and pave a new path. This process requires you to seek education about the complexity of obesity and then share your knowledge with your patients and colleagues. Lastly, you received tips on how to initiate time-efficient conversations.

In Chap. 5 you learned how to create an environment in which effective conversations can take place. You learned the importance of ensuring that the physical environment is safe, accessible, accommodating, comfortable, welcoming, and non-shaming. When this is not the case, it is another manifestation of weight bias, and contributes to patients delaying or avoiding healthcare. The need to create a positive emotional environment was stressed, as the language and practices of the office and clinical staff have a big impact on whether or not patients have a respectful, non-shaming experience. You learned that People First Language for obesity is the standard of care and that failure to use it demonstrates weight bias.

Chapter 6 provided you with a framework from which to initiate effective conversations. The value of building a respectful, collaborative partnership with your patients was emphasized, as was the need to keep the conversation focused on health. Motivational Interviewing (MI) provided you with guidance on how to elicit your patients' motivation, keep the conversation focused on your patients' goals, and honor your patients' autonomy. The 5As of obesity management provided you with a structure that will guide you through the process of initiating a discussion to arranging treatment in a manner that is patient-centered and keeps the therapeutic partnership intact. Guidance on how to select patients who will be most receptive to your message was provided.

In Chap. 7, clinical scenarios and conversations demonstrated how to start conversations in different practice settings with a variety of patients. Each scenario was followed by an explanation as to which strategies and principles were employed to build the clinician-patient relationship and move patients into treatment. These scenarios, and the explanations demonstrated how you can bring all of your knowledge into practice.

8.3 The Next Step

Now that you know how to initiate effective conversations with your patients, the next step is to educate them about obesity and guide them into treatment. If you will be providing your patients' obesity treatment, the next step is to schedule an obesity-specific history and physical appointment during which you will complete your comprehensive assessment and formulate a treatment plan. You may provide some or all components of treatment or refer to other clinicians, professionals, and community resources as needed. If you will not be providing treatment, appropriate referrals should be made.

8.4 Patient Education

When patients are considering treatment or are embarking on it, they need information about obesity and how it is managed. Whether or not you will be treating patients or referring them to other clinicians and resources, it is important to provide patients with an overview of their condition and how it is treated. If time permits, this can be discussed with the patient. If not, it is advisable to provide patient education materials that cover the elements discussed below. When discussion has taken place, patient education materials are still advisable as they reinforce what has been discussed with the clinician and provide patients with something to reference after the conversation. Education can be provided in the form of printed handouts, brochures, or be available on clinic websites.

Education should start with an introduction to the concept that obesity is a chronic health condition that requires a long-term treatment approach. Clinicians should explain the associated health risks and the benefits of a modest weight reduction of 5–10%, with attention to the specific health risks for the patient. Patients should be told that effective treatment is available and that they don't have to figure it out on their own. They should be informed that a thorough assessment will be performed, and a personalized plan will be given. Clinicians should frame the clinician-patient relationship as a partnership, reassure patients that all decisions will be made collaboratively, and that each element of the treatment plan will be implemented in a stepwise manner. The five comprehensive treatment modalities—nutrition, physical activity, behavioral counseling, pharmacotherapy, and bariatric surgery and procedures—should be introduced so that patients have an overview of the components of treatment. If bariatric surgery is being considered, patients should be informed that surgery is one aspect of treatment but that it doesn't replace the four pillars of nutrition, physical activity, behavioral counseling, and pharmacotherapy. They should be informed that appointments will be more frequent in the beginning in order to establish an effective treatment plan and to provide the support they need to implement and follow the plan, and that frequency will decrease when the condition stabilizes. It is important to reassure them that if challenges develop or relapses occur, appointment frequency will increase until stability is reestablished.

8.5   Obesity Treatment Options

As more clinicians recognize that obesity is a serious chronic condition, they are becoming educated on how to provide treatment in their current practice settings. Whether they are in primary or specialty care, they are finding ways to offer treatment that range from multi-disciplinary comprehensive models, to single clinicians providing all aspects of treatment, to coordinating treatment with other providers and resources. Although time, resources, and reimbursement for obesity treatment are limited in many practice settings, clinicians are finding creative ways to address obesity. While the situation in many practice settings is less than ideal, things are slowly improving. This section will provide you with information about the most common ways that treatment is provided.

Regardless of who is providing treatment, regular, obesity-specific appointments optimize outcomes. Although it is optimal to have a minimum of 16 appointments in the first year (1), this may not be possible for all patients. Appointment frequency may be limited by time, cost, clinician availability, treatment resources, transportation, and many other factors. When barriers preclude more frequent appointments, it is best to focus on regular follow-up, even if appointments can only occur once every 2–3 months.

8.5.1   Primary Care Settings

What can be accomplished in a primary care setting is dependent on time, resources, and other factors. Primary care providers who have completed additional obesity education integrate comprehensive obesity treatment into their primary care practices. They initiate conversations with appropriate patients during annual wellness visits, follow-up care, or when providing treatment for other conditions. When patients agree to treatment, these clinicians assist their patients in arranging it. Some have their patients return to see them for obesity-specific appointments that are integrated into their daily schedules. Others see their patients in comprehensive obesity treatment clinics that they operate one or more days per week within their practice setting. Some of these clinics are multi-disciplinary whereas others are staffed by a single clinician.

Some primary care clinicians manage obesity but refer patients to other healthcare professionals and community resources for some components of treatment. An example of this scenario is when a primary care clinician conducts a comprehensive obesity assessment, formulates a personalized treatment plan, and follows up regularly to manage the patient's response to treatment, prescribe and monitor anti-obesity medications, make any needed modifications to the treatment plan, and refers the patient for nutritional counseling, physical activity instruction, health coaching, or mental health counseling. Regardless of the practice model, if primary care clinicians are not getting an adequate response to treatment, they should refer their patients to an obesity specialist or bariatric surgery center.

Some primary care providers do not treat obesity but refer their patients to in-house clinicians and professionals who do. Those who do not have in-house resources refer their patients to outside clinicians and resources. See Table 8.1 for a list of potential referral sources. When referring patients to outside treatment, it is advisable to schedule follow-up in 2–6 months to ensure that the patient has accessed the treatment and is attending appointments regularly. This follow-up may be in the form of an appointment, phone call, or electronic communication. Any issues with access, follow-through, or other barriers can be addressed so that treatment can begin or resume.

8.5.2 Specialty Care Settings

Specialty care clinicians are increasingly incorporating obesity treatment into their practices. When treating the complications of obesity, they recognize that when obesity is treated first, the complications improve or resolve. For this reason, some offer comprehensive obesity treatment in their specialty care settings following

Table 8.1 Referral sources

Nutrition	Physical activity	Behavioral	Specialists
Dieticians	Physical therapists	Health coaches	Obesity specialists
Commercial weight loss programs	Exercise physiologists	Psychotherapists	Bariatric surgery centers
Cooking classes	Exercise trainers	Eating disorder specialists	
Community resources	Community programs & classes	Support groups	

similar models to those that take place in primary care. Examples of specialties that do so are endocrinology, obstetrics and gynecology, gastroenterology, orthopedics, cardiology, nephrology, sleep medicine, and rheumatology. If in-house obesity treatment is not available, they refer to obesity specialists and bariatric surgery centers.

8.5.3   Obesity Specialists

Obesity specialists may practice in primary and specialty care clinics or in separate obesity treatment clinics. These clinics may be independent or affiliated with a healthcare organization or hospital-based system. Some are multi-disciplinary and have obesity specialists, dieticians, health coaches, mental health professionals, and other types of providers on staff. In others, the clinicians deliver all components of comprehensive treatment. Some comprehensive obesity treatment centers have both non-surgical and surgical providers. Patients are evaluated and managed by obesity specialists and are referred to in-house surgical clinicians and surgeons for bariatric surgery but continue to be managed by the non-surgical specialists.

8.5.4   Bariatric Surgery Centers

Bariatric surgery centers offer multi-disciplinary surgical treatment. They are typically staffed with surgeons, nurse practitioners, physician assistants, registered nurses, dieticians, and mental health professionals, as well as clinical and office support staff. Some surgery centers have non-surgical obesity specialists who manage obesity prior to and after surgery and provide long-term obesity management.

Table 8.2 provides resources for locating clinicians who specialize in surgical and non-surgical obesity treatment.

Table 8.2 Resources for locating obesity specialists and bariatric surgery centers

Organization	Website link
American Society for Metabolic and Bariatric Surgery	https://asmbs.org/patients/find-a-provider
Obesity Action Coalition	https://obesitycareproviders.com/
Obesity Canada	https://locator.obesitycanada.ca/?_ga=2.24132794.1288463157.1609626881-1241536302.1608340333#!/
Obesity Medicine Association	https://obesitymedicine.org/find-obesity-treatment/

8.6   Summary

This book has prepared you to initiate productive conversations about obesity with your patients. Your knowledge of the seriousness of obesity and role of treatment in improving health, quality of life, and preventing complications will guide and inspire you to open the conversation. When you take the first step, it will lead you to the next and the next and the next. As your skills and confidence grow, you will find yourself opening the conversation earlier and more frequently. And as you do, you will watch your patients' health improve with each conversation.

Reference

1. Apovian CM, Aronne LJ, Bessesen DH, McDonnell ME, Murad MH, Pagotto U, et al. Pharmacological management of obesity: an endocrine society clinical practice guideline. J Clin Endocrinol Metab. 2015;100(2):342–62.